Therapy for Adults Molested as Children

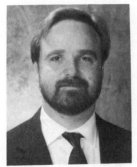

John Briere, PhD, is Associate Professor in the Departments of Psychiatry and Psychology at the University of Southern California School of Medicine, and a clinical psychologist at the Department of Emergency Psychiatric Services of LAC-USC Medical Center. He is author or editor of five books, two psychological tests, and numerous articles in the areas of child abuse, psychological trauma, and interpersonal violence. Dr. Briere is on the editorial boards of several scholarly journals and is on the board of directors of the American Professional Society on the Abuse of Children (APSAC) and the International Society for Traumatic Stress Studies (ISTSS). He consults to local, national, and international agencies on the topics of trauma, violence, and research methodology, and regularly presents workshops on the assessment and treatment of psychological trauma.

Therapy for Adults Molested as Children

Beyond Survival

Revised and Expanded Edition

JOHN BRIERE

SPRINGER PUBLISHING COMPANY

Springer Publishing Company, Inc.
536 Broadway
New York, NY 10012-3955

96 97 98 99 00 / 5 4 3 2 1

Library of Congress Cataloging-in-Publication Data

Briere, John.
    Therapy for adults molested as children : beyond survival / John
Briere. — Rev. and expanded.
        p.   cm.
    Includes bibliographical references and index.
    ISBN 0-8261-5641-X
    1. Adult child sexual abuse victims—Mental health.
2. Psychotherapy.   I. Title.
RC569.5.A28B75   1996
616.85'83690651—dc20   96-8221
                                                                   CIP

Printed in the United States of America

Contents

Foreword

It is an honor to have been invited to write the foreword to the second edition of *Therapy for Adults Molested as Children*. I have long been an admirer of Dr. John Briere. He is an individual of integrity as well as a productive scholar and gifted clinician. Throughout his career, Dr. Briere has been dedicated to learning and teaching about adults abused as children. He has advanced professional knowledge of the characteristics and needs of this population through numerous research studies and publications and has used this knowledge to develop an innovative model of treatment. This model was first published in 1989; in this second edition, it is substantially revised and updated. In addition to describing the theory and strategy for the treatment of adult survivors, it offers sound clinical guidance for a wide variety of process and content issues that tend to emerge during this therapy.

In recent years, both the prevalence and the toll of child sexual abuse have been acknowledged as never before. The sexual abuse of children is alarmingly prevalent in North America, its aftereffects diverse and tenacious. Sexual abuse, especially when incestuous or otherwise occurring within an established relationship where sexual contact is proscribed, is now recognized as a traumatic stressor with high potential for post-traumatic consequences at the time of the abuse and later in life. Its occurrence in childhood (and often

over the course of childhood) has major developmental implications: the child's psychosexual, physical, and interpersonal development is compromised resulting in an idiosyncratic pattern of
developmental delays, fixations, and/or accelerations. These effects
have often been ascribed diagnoses that, in effect, blame the victim
for her reactions without an adequate understanding of their origin.
New diagnostic conceptualizations are now emerging that take
abuse as well as developmental impact into account.

The adult survivor of sexual abuse who seeks treatment often
does so without having received either acknowledgment or help at
the time of the abuse or subsequently. He or she presents with a
diverse array of post-traumatic, affective, characterological, and relational issues at least partially derived from the abuse that have likely
compounded over time. Thus, the clinician is presented with what
is often a formidable treatment challenge of numerous symptoms
and a client whose self and relationship capacities were influenced
and distorted by exploitation. An unfortunate complication is the
fact that most practicing clinicians (even the most recent graduates)
have had little or no formal training in identifying and treating postabuse trauma as part of their professional education. Complicating
the matter even more is the controversy currently surrounding the
treatment of adults who report a history of abuse. Critics allege that
therapists are behaving irresponsibly by naively overbelieving their
clients' accounts of abuse or, worse yet, are suggesting and creating
false memories of abuse as an explanation of their clients' symptoms.

This work was originally published as a sourcebook to guide clinicians in their treatment of abuse survivors. This second edition
builds upon the first and provides additional direction, much
needed during this time of controversy and as large numbers of
adults reporting abuse histories continue to seek treatment. In the
first part of the book, research-based information about the lasting
effects of sexual abuse is presented. These effects are discussed not
only as symptoms but in a more conceptually sophisticated way as
multi-faceted core issues. A discussion of the philosophy of treatment follows. Dr. Briere advocates an abuse-focused perspective
from which to understand the client and orient the treatment; however, this approach is not free-standing and is presented along with

other therapeutic perspectives, grounded in the established tenets of psychotherapeutic practice. One of the major strengths of this book is its integrationist approach—a traumatic stress perspective is blended with psychodynamic, object relations, self-psychology, and cognitive-behavioral perspectives and strategies. Additionally, the therapy is oriented towards moving the client beyond victimization towards personal growth and improved functioning.

Dr. Briere is careful to note that an abuse-focused perspective does not mean that the therapist is solely oriented towards abuse and trauma-related issues to the exclusion of all others. Rather, this perspective holds that abuse can have a profound impact on current psychological functioning that must not be minimized or negated but instead must be recognized and worked with. The remainder of the book addresses some of the most common and vexing technical, relational, and process issues in the treatment of this population. These are some of the issues most often implicated in ineffective or problematic treatment, the very issues that the therapist was most likely not trained to anticipate, recognize, or work with. These include management of the treatment frame, traumatic transference and countertransference issues (including those that are specifically gender-related), common abuse-related issues and reenactments, assessment and treatment planning related to traumatic symptoms, sequencing, stabilization before uncovering, and titration to the client's emotional capacity and tolerance. Special attention is given to technical aspects of work with incomplete/dissociated/repressed memory. The clinician is advised to maintain a position of neutrality especially with those clients who struggle with uncertainty about their history yet to be open to the possibility of unremembered or partially remembered abuse as well as to the client's pain.

The final chapter is devoted to a discussion of the impact of therapy of adult survivors on the clinician. Although this therapy can be very satisfying, it holds an unusually high number of challenges and pitfalls. It can result in overidentification and rescuing, burnout and abandonment, and even revictimization by the uninformed or misguided therapist. These and other difficulties that attend this work are now supplemented by anxieties generated by the false memory controversy. Therapists must stay informed about new developments in this rapidly changing field, must monitor personal reactions, burn-out, and self-care issues, and must engage in continuing education and consultation for informed clinical practice. This book provides a foundation of essential information for this work, updated to include recent developments and advances in the field. It admirably achieves its stated goal of advancing the treatment of adult survivors of abuse and supports the therapist in this most important endeavor.

CHRISTINE A. COURTOIS, PhD
Psychologist, Private Practice
Director of Clinical Training
THE CENTER: Post-traumatic &
Dissociative Disorders Program
The Psychatric Institute of Washington

Acknowledgments

I would like to thank all of those who assisted me, in one manner or another, with the second edition of this book. These include Rod Shaner, M.D., and Rita Ruiz for their continuing support of my academic endeavors, Diana Elliott, Ph.D., for her voluminous clinical and research input, Don Putnam and Susan Killison for friendship and assistance, especially at a critical juncture (when are you coming back to LA?), Bill Tucker and Louise Farkas at Springer Publishing Company for their editorial and technical assistance, and Cheryl Lanktree, Ph.D. for partnership, inspiration, and patience.

Introduction

This book, substantially expanded and revised in its second edition, is intended to be a sourcebook on the treatment of adults molested as children. The need for detailed and up-to-date information on the assessment and treatment of sexual abuse survivors remains clear. Modern general population surveys suggest that about one third of women and one sixth of men in North America report sexually victimization that occurred during or before their midteens (Finkelhor, Hotaling, Lewis, & Smith, 1989; Peters, Wyatt, & Finkelhor, 1986; Russell, 1983b). Other studies report that more than one half of teenage and adult prostitutes have histories of childhood sexual abuse and that similar numbers of substance abusers were sexually abused as children (Bagley & Young, 1987: Briere & Runtz, 1987). Even more relevant to mental health workers are the results of research indicating that between 40% and 70% of women requesting psychotherapy or psychiatric services report having been sexually abused during childhood (Briere, 1992a). As presented in chapter 1, most of these studies indicate that childhood sexual abuse is associated with serious long-term psychological harm, including poor self-esteem, posttraumatic stress, depression, substance abuse, sexual problems, interpersonal difficulties, and self-injurious behaviors.

Because of the relative recency of clinical interest in sexual abuse,

1

most mental health professionals have had little formal training in recognizing or treating post–sexual-abuse trauma (Alpert & Paulson, 1990; Enns, McNeilly, Corkery, & Gilbert, 1995; Pope & Felman-Summers, 1992). This relative dearth of training has been emphasized recently by critics of abuse-focused therapy. These individuals suggest that inept and ill-trained clinicians frequently use misguided therapeutic techniques that create or distort memories of abuse in their clients. Although extremist views on this subject are questioned on several occasions in this book, it is clear that a central premise of this critique has some validity: Not all clinicians are providing helpful or appropriate interventions regarding abuse trauma, and some interventions are likely to be harmful. Like any other area requiring specialized training, abuse-relevant therapy can be misapplied by those with inadequate technical preparation and clinical experience, sometimes resulting in malpractice and negative outcomes.

Other clinicians err in the opposite direction: overlooking or minimizing their clients' sexual abuse histories, and applying therapeutic techniques that, at best, do not address abuse trauma. Like their cohorts on the "other side," these individuals may reveal their lack of training or understanding of abuse-related trauma by adhering to extreme positions regarding child abuse and its effects (or lack thereof). Both groups require further education if they are to be helpful with sexual abuse survivors.

The first edition of this book has been substantially revised in response to this continuing gap in mental health training and practice. This edition also includes more complex and technical information that will be of interest to the experienced trauma therapist. Chapter 1 summarizes several decades of research on the long-term effects of sexual victimization. Chapter 2 outlines traditional psychiatric views of these effects, primarily as they relate to diagnoses of "hysteria" and "borderline personality disorder," and describes the recently raised notion of a "false memory syndrome." Chapter 3 offers an integrated theory of postabuse symptom development and suggests that certain "core" phenomena account for many of the psychosocial difficulties associated with a childhood history of sexual victimization. Subsequent chapters delineate an overall philosophy of treatment and outline a model of therapeutic intervention that can be helpful in treating especially severe sexual abuse trauma. Finally, the impact of this work on the therapist is discussed, and potential remedies are presented.

Throughout this book the reader will encounter descriptions or interventions that are relevant to individuals who were not sexually abused as children, but who experienced other types of abusive childhood experiences, such as physical or psychological maltreatment or emotional neglect. This overlap in presenting problems is not surprising because the child's experience of any form of victimization is bound to include common feelings of confusion, fear, helplessness, and betrayal, and may motivate the development of similar long-term coping strategies. The general focus of this book is not, therefore, to the exclusion of other ways in which children can be hurt in our society. As common as is sexual abuse, physical and emotional cruelty may be even more frequent, and are probably equally injurious in certain areas of functioning.

This second edition of *Therapy for Adults Molested as Children* also reflects newer ideas my colleagues and I have developed regarding etiology, phenomenology, and treatment. I have increased considerably the material devoted to "self" issues in sexual abuse trauma, with special attention to issues involving identity, boundary, and affect regulation. A theory of intrusive symptomatology as emotional processing is introduced, and the implications of this model for therapeutic intervention are discussed. Gender-related differences in abuse trauma are described at greater length, especially with reference to the impacts of sex-role socialization on the development of affect regulation problems in male survivors. In addition, some of the notions I introduced in the first edition regarding the adaptive components of "self-destructive" acts have been expanded in terms of a more formal theory of tension reduction. The chapter on transference and countertransference also has been expanded, including the presentation of several identifiable transferential patterns frequently present in abuse-related psychotherapy. Finally, the behavioral techniques of graduated exposure, habituation, and counterconditioning have been more formally described and integrated into the therapeutic approach presented here, based on their clear relevance to the treatment of trauma-related symptomatology.

For obvious ethical reasons, all case histories and client quotations presented in this book have been disguised and cannot be traced back to any one individual. Among other alterations, the demographic characteristics of the various clients described have been randomly combined or altered.

Although this is a considerably more technical book than the first edition, it maintains the philosophical perspective present in that version: that sexual abuse is, in part, a social act, with social ramifications, requiring social—as well as psychological—remedies.

The Lasting Effects of Sexual Abuse

1

I dreamed I was in a war, like my brother was. I was trying to escape and people were shooting at me. I get away to a safe place, on a hill or something. And I start crying because I'm safe. I can't believe I got away without being shot. And then I look down, and I'm bleeding. I thought I was safe, but I was shot. And I didn't even know it. I got away, but here I am, still bleeding. (Male sexual abuse survivor)

For those who have experienced sexual abuse, or have listened objectively to someone who has, there is little doubt that such experiences can be harmful. In fact, one is initially struck with the bizarreness of child molestation. Could anyone really do that to a child? How must it feel to know that your father or mother or teacher did such a thing? And what would it be like to live with that? With them? As therapists, we hear of violation and betrayal; we listen to the rage, sorrow, and self-hatred. The damage sometimes seems immense, perhaps beyond our abilities to help.

Yet, ironically, there is controversy among some authorities as to whether sexual abuse even produces negative effects. Not that long ago, a noted psychiatrist wrote that "research is inconclusive as to the psychological harmfulness of incestuous behavior" (Henderson, 1983, p. 34). More recently, another prominent psychiatrist questioned whether "a sexual encounter between an adult and a child—no matter how short, no matter how tender, loving, and non-painful—automatically

and predictably must be psychologically traumatic to the child" (Gardner, 1992, p. 191): a scenario that says as much about the author's view
of sexual abuse as it does his conclusions about its potential effects. Others have suggested that many sexual abuse reports reflect false allegations, false memory syndrome, or some combination of therapist
incompetence and client avarice in the context of wrongly prosecuted
civil litigation (Loftus & Ketcham, 1994; Ofshe & Watters, 1994; Wakefield & Underwager, 1993).

This book takes a position that is generally at odds with such notions,
although it does not overlook the fact that both clients and therapists are
vulnerable to the vagaries of the human condition. As this chapter
shows, most published studies indicate that sexual abuse is commonly
(although not inevitably) associated with significant psychological pain
and suffering—trauma that may persist over the years unless specifically resolved. In one review of this literature, for example, Browne and
Finkelhor (1986a, 1986b) describe the findings of 52 studies on the
impact of childhood sexual abuse and conclude that "empirical studies
with adults confirm many of the long-term effects of sexual abuse mentioned in the clinical literature." They further note that "the risk of initial and long-term mental health impairment for victims of child sexual
abuse should be taken very seriously" (1986a, p. 72). Other, more recent
reviews offer similar conclusions (Briere & Runtz, 1993; Finkelhor, 1990;
Neumann, Houskamp, Pollock, & Briere, 1996).

The purpose of this chapter is to acquaint the reader with those
types of psychological distress commonly associated with post–
sexual-abuse trauma. Because of the many problems reported in the
abuse literature, the known results of sexual victimization will be
divided here somewhat arbitrarily into four major kinds of psychological effects. These categories, which often coexist in the sexual
abuse survivor, are referred to as (a) posttraumatic stress, (b) cognitive effects, (c) emotional effects, and (d) interpersonal effects. Each
category is described in detail and relevant research is cited.

POSTTRAUMATIC STRESS

The term *posttraumatic stress disorder* (PTSD) is typically used to
describe the psychological experience of certain war veterans, survivors of major earthquakes, rape victims, and other people who

have experienced severe trauma. In this regard, PTSD refers to those characteristic psychological reactions that frequently follow disaster, victimization, or other events capable of producing extreme psychological stress (Astin, Layne, Camilleri, & Foy, 1994; Saigh, 1992). According to the American Psychiatric Association's *Diagnostic and Statistical Manual of Mental Disorders,* fourth edition (DSM-IV), a combination of the following criteria must be met for a diagnosis of PTSD:

1. The existence of an event that involved witnessing or experiencing actual or threatened death or serious injury, or a threat to physical integrity of self or others, that produced intense fear, helplessness, or horror. Childhood sexual abuse is specifically included in this criterion, despite the fact that not all abuse confers threat of death or injury.
2. Later reexperiencing or recollecting the trauma in one's mind—for example, through recurrent dreams of the stressor or "flashbacks" (intrusive sensory memories) to the original traumatic situation; or an intensification of symptoms on exposure to situations that resemble the original traumatic event.
3. Persistent avoidance of stimuli associated with the event and numbing of responsiveness to the external world—for example, dissociation, withdrawal, inability to recall important aspects of the trauma, restricted affect, or loss of interest in daily events.
4. Persistent symptoms of increased arousal, not present before the trauma, such as sleep disturbance, irritability, difficulty concentrating, hypervigilance to danger in the environment, and an exaggerated startle response.

Several writers have suggested that sexual abuse during childhood, perhaps especially within the family, may produce posttraumatic symptoms, both immediately and later in life (Donaldson & Gardner, 1985; Gold, Milan, Mayall, & Johnson, 1994; Goodwin, 1984; Greenwald & Leitenberg, 1990; Lindberg & Distad, 1985a; Rowan, Foy, Rodriguez, & Ryan, 1994; Saunders, Villeponteaux, Lipovsky, Kilpatrick, & Veronen, 1992).[1] McLeer, Deblinger, Atkins,

---

[1]At first glance, changes to the PTSD criteria in DSM-IV appear to make it more difficult to assign this diagnosis to child abuse survivors because the new criteria (inappropriately, I believe) require threat of death or serious injury. DSM-III and III-R did not limit traumatic events solely to physical (as opposed to psychological) danger. However, DSM-IV makes a special exception that sexually abused children can develop PTSD in response to their molestation, even if there was no threat of death or injury. As a result, the diagnosis of chronic PTSD in adult survivors is still appropriate in DSM-IV

Foa, and Raphe (1988), for example, reported that more than one half of the sexually abused children they studied met DSM-III-R criteria for PTSD. Similarly, Briere, Elliott, Harris, and Cotman (1995) report that sexual abuse survivors in inpatient or outpatient therapy have significantly higher scores on the Anxious Arousal, Intrusive Experiences, and Defensive Avoidance scales of the Trauma Symptom Inventory (Briere, 1995)—data supporting the probability of posttraumatic stress in at least some of these subjects (see Appendix 1 of this book for further information on this sample). In fact, a review of the sexual abuse literature emphasizes the appropriateness of viewing severe post–sexual-abuse trauma as, in part, a complex form of PTSD (Briere, in press, b). As the following discussion shows, each of the criteria for PTSD has been described in the literature as a long-term effect of childhood sexual abuse.

A Traumatic Event That Involved Intense Fear, Helplessness, or Horror

Sexual abuse is defined in this book as actual sexual contact with a child that either (a) is accomplished by force or threat of force, regardless of the ages of the participants, or (b) involves an adult and a child, regardless of whether there is deception or the child understands the sexual nature of the activity (Berliner & Elliott, 1996). Although most research definitions require that the child be younger than 15 or 16 years of age and that the abuser be 5 or more years older, most cases appear to involve more obvious age disparities, typically children younger than 12 years of age and men in their mid-20s or older (Finkelhor, 1979a; Russell, 1986).

The minimal "sexual contact" requirement is often grossly exceeded: In one random clinical example of 133 female sexual abuse victims (Briere, 1988), 43% reported incest by a parent or stepparent, 77% had been penetrated orally, anally, or vaginally, and 56% were also physically abused. Of this sample, 17% reported especially bizarre abuse, including multiple simultaneous perpetrators, insertion of foreign objects, ritualistic abuse, or torture. Similarly, of the 60% of adolescent mothers who reported childhood sexual abuse in an Illinois study (Ounce of Prevention Fund, 1987), 33% reported having been raped by one or more abusers, and 25% reported attempted rape. More than 25% of these women had been abused on 10 or more occasions by the same person. It should be noted that such samples typically represent examples of more severe sexual victimization relative to, for instance, the average abuse experiences of university students, professionals, or other higher functioning groups (Elliott & Briere, 1992; Fromuth, 1985). Nevertheless, data from clinical samples alert us to the extreme level of intrusion and violence that can accompany childhood sexual victimization.

Although early writers often sought to downplay the aversive quality and impact of such abuse, most modern researchers acknowledge that sexual victimization is a frightening, painful, and psychologically overwhelming experience for many children (see, however, Wakefield and Underwager's seemingly pro-pedophilia interview in Paidika [1993] and Gardner's [1992] remarks regarding abuse "hysteria" for contrary positions). Regarding the intrusiveness of sexual abuse, Finkelhor (1979a) found that of 530 university women, 58% of those sexually abused as children described reacting to victimization with fear, and 26% stated they experienced "shock." In a community sample of 930 women, Russell (1986) found that 80% of those who had been abused were "somewhat" to "extremely" upset, and that 78% reported long-term negative effects of the abuse experience. Later analysis indicated that long-term psychological trauma was especially likely when incest victims had experienced severe victimization, for example, oral/anal/vaginal penetration, abuse occurring over an extended period, or especially violent abuse (Herman, Russell, & Trocki, 1986). The presence of such data in nonclinical groups (i.e., in individuals not requesting help for psychological problems) underlines the traumagenic qualities of sexual abuse.

Reexperiencing of the Trauma

Many survivors of childhood sexual victimization describe intrusive memories of or flashbacks to the abuse, as well as recurring nightmares (Elliott & Briere, 1995; Lindberg & Distad, 1985a; Meiselman, 1990; Rowan, Foy, Rodriquez, & Ryan, 1994). These reexperiencing phenomena represent, in part, classically conditioned recollections of the original abuse event(s) that are triggered by reminiscent stimuli in the survivor's current environment (a more functional component of this phenomenon is also presented in chapter 6). Abuse-related flashbacks can involve all of the senses, such that the survivor may experience sudden visual, auditory, olfactory, gustatory, or tactile memories of the assault. Flashbacks may manifest, for example, as briefly feeling someone's hands on one's inner thigh, seeing one's perpetrator's genitalia or angry face, hearing sexual comments, smelling stale sweat or alcohol, or tasting semen. These periods of reliving the abuse can be so sudden and compelling as to produce a temporary break with the current environment, resulting in what may be misinterpreted as hallucinations or psychosis (Gelinas, 1983).

The nightmares of adolescents and adults who were victimized as children may involve a variety of events and images, although a few themes are especially common. Probably the most frequent are dreams that replay actual scenes from the molestation, in what have been referred to as "Type 1" nightmares (Briere, 1992a). These may be graphically realistic or may be elaborations or variations on the original experience. Others (i.e., Type 2 nightmares) are more symbolic in nature, involving, for example, shadowy, threatening figures by one's bed, attacks by coiling snakes or snarling monsters, frightening pursuits down dark halls or alleys, or gory mutilation or disfigurement. Typical in these scenes, regardless of manifest content, are feelings of terror and helplessness—sometimes presented as the dreamer being paralyzed or in some way unable to escape.[2] In light of the power of posttraumatic nightmares (Hartmann, 1984), it is not surprising, as is mentioned later, that many sexual abuse survivors experience chronic sleep disturbance.

The last intrusive PTSD phenomenon relevant to sexual abuse survivors is complex reexperiencing: the contemporaneous triggering of early abuse memories and emotions of such intensity that the survivor may believe he or she is suddenly back in childhood, undergoing abuse again. Common triggers of reexperiencing are

---

[2]Although sexual abuse survivors often report such nightmares, it does not follow that all nightmares with equivalent content indicate the presence of sexual abuse. Violent and highly disturbing nightmares may arise from a variety of sources, of which child sexual abuse is only one.

sexual interactions (Jehu & Gazan, 1983); exploitation by a more powerful person or persons (Briere, 1992a); physical violation or assault; and, in some cases, first disclosures of having been sexually abused as a child. In many instances, the immediate result of complex reexperiencing is a dissociative episode or a period of panic, depression, or withdrawal.

Numbing of General Responsiveness

This component of PTSD refers to an attenuation in feeling or emotion, wherein the individual experiences reduced reactivity, detachment from others, or constricted emotionality. Several clinicians have noted the prevalence of these problems among sexual abuse survivors (Courtois, 1988; Gil, 1988; Meiselman, 1990), as have researchers of sexual abuse effects. This coping strategy is thought to develop during the victimization process, when any means of avoiding acute pain, fear, and humiliation is reinforced. This avoidance defense may then generalize to other aversive and anxiety-provoking experiences later in life, eventually becoming a relatively autonomous and pervasive symptom.

> Alice, a 19-year-old woman is brought to the emergency room by her roommate, who states that she has been "zoned out" for nearly 24 hours: not eating, not responding to conversation, and "just looking at the wall." During her interview, Alice's eyes are fixed and staring, and her face is blank. She responds to questions in a monosyllabic, distracted manner, denying hallucinations or recent drug use. When told that she might be admitted to the hospital, she states to the psychologist, without perceptible emotion, "If you're going to hurt me, I don't want to know about it, OK?" This will be Alice's third hospitalization, the first of which followed a suicide attempt at age 12, prompted by her father's imprisonment for molesting Alice, her sister, and a friend.

At its most basic level, reduced responsiveness is a form of dissociation. Various studies of sexual abuse survivors (Anderson, Yasenik, & Ross, 1993; Briere & Conte, 1993; Briere & Runtz, 1990a; Chu & Dill, 1990; Gold et al., 1994) report a constellation of dissociative symptoms, such as cognitive disengagement from the environment into a seemingly neutral state ("spacing out"), derealization (the experience that things around one are false or unreal), depersonalization (the sense that one is different from one's usual self), out-of-body experiences (often involving the sensation of floating outside of one's body and traveling elsewhere), and circumscribed blanks in otherwise continuous memory. Dissociation may be described as a defensive disruption in the normally occurring connections among feelings, thoughts, behaviors, and memories, consciously or unconsciously invoked to reduce psychological distress (Briere, 1992).

Of special relevance to abuse survivors is the posttraumatic symptom of impaired recall, referred to in DSM-IV as dissociative amnesia. Although the entire notion of posttraumatic amnesia has been questioned by some (Loftus, 1993), memory disturbance in some former sexual abuse victims has been described by several researchers in the area (Briere & Conte, 1993; Elliott & Briere, 1995; Feldman-Summers & Pope, 1994; Herman & Schatzow, 1987; Loftus, Polonsky, & Fullilove, 1994; Williams, 1994), primarily involving some level of self-reported amnesia for the original abuse experience. As chapters 2 and 7 indicate, such motivated forgetting of childhood events is likely to be a powerful dissociative defense against integrated reexperiencing of the trauma and pain of victimization—sometimes producing complete lack of memory for extended periods of childhood, but more typically resulting in incomplete or partial memories of painful events.

The frequency of such experiences in the sexual abuse survivor suggests that dissociation may represent a powerful defense against abuse-related memories or feelings. Whether such symptoms occur as components of PTSD, or exist in relative isolation as a dissociative disorder, they appear to function as a way for the victim to state that "this isn't actually happening" (derealization), "it isn't happening to me" (depersonalization), or "it never happened to me" (amnesia). Perhaps the most dramatic example of this dissociation from abusive events is that of dissociative identity disorder or "multiple personalities" ("it happened to somebody else"), typically linked by researchers to (among other factors) sexual abuse trauma (Coons & Milstein, 1986; Putnam, 1989; Ross, 1989). Because of its special relevance to post–sexual-abuse trauma and its frequent impact on therapy, dissociation is addressed at considerable length in chapters 2, 3, and 6.

Autonomic Hyperarousal

As mentioned earlier, PTSD often involves a variety of other symptoms, including sleep disturbance, difficulties in maintaining concentration, hyperalertness, and irritability. Just as many of these symptoms are found in rape victims (Burgess & Holmstrom, 1974; Elliott & Mok, 1995; Koss & Harvey, 1991) and other victims of trauma (van der Kolk, 1987), sexual abuse survivors are likely to experience similar difficulties at some point in their lives.

Such autonomic hyperarousal often presents cognitively as extreme alertness to the possibility of danger. This hypervigilance may, paradoxically, coexist with an inability to concentrate for extended periods, producing an individual who is constantly scanning the environment but who may have difficulty focusing her or his attention when needed. Although only scantily documented in the sexual abuse literature, such chronic arousal appears to be most common among victims of especially severe sexual abuse, many of whom have also been physically maltreated in childhood. Continual hyperarousal may produce physical difficulties ranging from headaches and hypertension to back pain and gastrointestinal problems (Briere, 1992c).

Sleep disturbance (involving insomnia, restless sleep, nightmares, and midsleep or early morning awakenings) is a common result of abuse-related hyperarousal. Researchers, such as Sedney and Brooks (1984) and Briere and Runtz (1987), report that sexual abuse survivors are approximately twice as likely as nonabused individuals to have sleep problems of some sort. Chronic hyperarousal can delay the onset of sleep and cause sleep to become more shallow, resulting in restlessness and proneness to awakening. More psychodynamically, it is clear that sleep is experienced by the survivor as a time of maximal vulnerability, when vigilance and defenses are at their lowest and when frightening dreams are likely. This sense of helplessness is compounded by the likelihood that the abuse (especially if it was incest) occurred in darkness or in the bedroom.

We can understand, then, when sexual abuse survivors in therapy report that "nighttime is the worst time."

COGNITIVE EFFECTS

In addition to PTSD effects, it is clear that child abuse, including molestation, can alter the way the victim perceives and understands herself, others, and the future (Janoff-Bulman, 1992; Jehu, 1989; Jehu, Klassen, & Gazan, 1985–86; McCann, Pearlman, Sackheim, & Abrahamson, 1988). Cognitive theorists have shown that similar distortions can be the basis for severe affective changes, such as clinical depression and the anxiety disorders (Beck, 1967; Beck, Emory, & Greenberg, 1985). The most common abuse-related cognitive alterations appear to be (a) negative self-evaluation and guilt, (b) perceived helplessness and hopelessness, and (c) distrust of others.

Negative Self-Evaluation and Guilt

It is not uncommon for sexual abuse survivors to see themselves as bad, evil, unintelligent, or unattractive, as well as generally responsible for their unhappiness and pain. As Herman (1981) noted of her group of adults sexually abused as children, "with depressing regularity, these women referred to themselves as bitches, witches, and whores" (p. 97). In an examination of the cognitive distortions found in former sexual abuse victims, Jehu, Gazan, and Klassen (1984–85) found that more than 50% of their female sample endorsed statements, such as " I am worthless and bad"; "No man could care for me without a sexual relationship"; "I am inferior to others because I did not have normal experiences"; and "I must have been seductive and provocative when I was young." In agreement with the findings of Jehu et al., several clinicians report that sexual abuse survivors present with clinically significant levels of impaired self-esteem (Courtois, 1979a, 1988; Herman, 1981; Mendel, 1995; Salter, 1995).

Roger is a blind, 28-year-old man originally came to his local community mental health center requesting help with relationships. Over time, he reveals involvement in sadomasochistic sexual practices, wherein he inevitably acts in the passive role. When asked if this is what he wants, Roger admits that "I really don't care for the sex that much." He appears unconcerned, however, about the dangers that he faces as a blind person who is habitually tied up, beaten, and violated. He later describes feelings of self-hatred and self-disgust, and reports a sense of calm when he is being "punished." Roger's childhood includes extensive sexual torture from age 6 to 13 at the hands of at least two older brothers.

There are several reasons for the negative self-evaluation of sexual abuse survivors. First, as noted by Symonds (1975), there is often a "marked reluctance and resistance of society to accept the innocence or accidental nature of victim behavior" (p. 19)—a skepticism that is frequently communicated to the survivor. Society's tendency to blame the victim impacts on him or her in a variety of ways, as discussed subsequently. Equally disturbing, however, is the victim's tendency to blame herself for having been injured or hurt regardless of the circumstance (Janoff-Bulman & Frieze, 1983; Miller & Porter, 1983). This phenomenon appears to involve what have been described as "just world" beliefs (Lerner, 1980). Lerner notes that "people want to and have to believe [that] they live in a just world so they can go about their daily lives with a sense of trust, hope, and confidence in their future" (p. 14). The victim may choose to believe that "I got what I deserved" as opposed to the potentially more frightening notion that violence is random and unjust, and that one cannot do things to avoid being victimized. Thus, in addition to its negative effects, self-blame may serve as a defense against feelings of total powerlessness for some victims (Lamb, 1986; Wortman, 1976).

Although the mechanisms cited previously produce an element of self-blame and subsequent self-derogation in victims of many forms of violence, there appear to be specific aspects of childhood sexual abuse that yield especially negative self-perceptions. As noted by Sandra Butler (1978), there is often a "conspiracy of silence" surrounding sexual abuse, invoked both by the abuser in the interests of self-protection and the reactions of society to abuse disclosures. Such secrecy conveys to the abuse victim the notion that she or he was involved in a shameful act and was, in fact, a guilty coconspirator. This process, which Finkelhor and associates (1986) call "stigmatization," includes

> the negative connotations—for example, badness, shame, and guilt—
> that are communicated to the child about the [abuse] experiences and
> then become incorporated into the child's self image. . . . They can
> come directly from the abuser, who may blame the victim for the
> activity, denigrate the victim, or, simply through his furtiveness, con-
> vey a sense of shame about the behavior. (p. 184)

As Finkelhor notes, it is, therefore, not surprising that many sexual abuse survivors report guilt and shame related to their victimization. These negative esteem effects on the sexual abuse victim tend to generalize and elaborate over time, producing in many cases chronic self-hatred and self-destructiveness (McCann et al., 1988).

Helplessness and Hopelessness

Because of the violation and "temporary loss of all personal choice" (Terr, 1985, p. 821) that accompanies many instances of child abuse, sexual abuse survivors often experience pervasive feelings of helplessness and hopelessness. Many aspects of sexual victimization are antithetic to feelings of personal power or self-efficacy. As noted by Finkelhor and associates (1986), these include (a) the child's experience of invasion of her or his body by a hurtful (or at least coercive) person; (b) the often repetitive nature of incest and other types of sexual victimization, resulting in chronic feelings of vulnerability and inability to protect oneself from danger; and (c) the experience of many victims that their abuse disclosures are not believed by others, despite their best efforts.

Together, these abuse dynamics reinforce to the survivor that she is relatively powerless in the face of adversity or negative events. This learned helplessness may be at the root of several behaviors and reactions found in many sexually abused individuals, including susceptibility to later victimization by others, passivity, and basic perception of self as "victim" (Peterson & Seligman, 1983). As is described later, such feelings of helplessness and hopelessness, in combination with low self-esteem and (in some survivors) difficulties with affect modulation, may also produce negative mood states—perhaps most notably clinical depression.

Distrust of Others

Having discovered at an early age that safety is not guaranteed and that betrayal can occur at any moment, many sexual abuse victims become preoccupied with what might be described as "the reality of danger." As Terr (1985) notes in a more general context: "Traumatized children so sharply fear many directly trauma-related and mundane items that they demonstrate massive interferences with optimism and trust" (p. 820). Although this dynamic may result in pervasive feelings of anxiety and fear, as described subsequently, there are also interpersonal impacts of betrayal and experienced lack of safety (McCann et al., 1988; Perloff, 1983). As Finkelhor (1987) notes: "[Abused] children discover that someone on whom they were vitally dependent has caused them or wishes to cause them harm" (p.15), a lesson that can easily generalize to later distrust of others (Courtois, 1988; Herman, 1992; Meiselman, 1978, 1990; Tsai & Wagner, 1978), expectations of injustice, and pervasive anger—especially toward individuals of the same gender as their abuser (Courtois, 1979a, 1988; Peters, 1976; Russell, 1986). As the treatment sections of this book indicate, this lack of trust and sometimes seemingly inexhaustible depot of rage can have real implications for psychotherapy with sexual abuse survivors.

EMOTIONAL EFFECTS

Anxiety

Elevated anxiety has been documented as overrepresented among adults who were sexually abused as children (Hunter, 1991; Murphy et al., 1988; Runtz, 1987; Yama, Tovey, & Fogas, 1993). Clinical experience suggests that adults with histories of child sexual abuse frequently present with cognitive, conditioned, and somatic components of anxiety. As would be predicted by Beck and Emery's (1985) model of anxiety disorder, cognitive aspects of abuse-related anxiety seems typically to involve (a) a hypervigilance to danger in the environment, (b) preoccupation with control, and (c) misinterpretation of neutral or positive interpersonal stimuli (e.g., intimacy and relatedness) as evidence of threat or danger.

The conditioned components of adult abuse-specific anxiety reside in the fact that child sexual abuse usually occurs in human relationships where closeness and nurturance is expected, yet intrusion, abandonment, devaluation, or pain occur. As a result, a classically conditioned association may form between various social or environmental stimuli and danger, such that a variety of interpersonal events (e.g., relationships and social situations) elicit fear (Wheeler & Berliner, 1988). This conditioned anxiety may also manifest as sexual dysfunction when sexual stimuli become linked with danger or pain during the sexual abuse process. Meiselman (1978), for example, found that 87% of her clinical sample of sexual abuse survivors had "serious" sexual problems compared with 20% of those not sexually abused in childhood. Similarly, Maltz and Holman (1987) report that 60% of their group of incest survivors experienced pain during intercourse, and 46% were anorgasmic. The frequency of which other studies find increased sexual dysfunction among abuse survivors (Becker, Skinner, Abel, & Treacy, 1982; Courtois, 1979a; Finkelhor, 1979a; Wyatt, Newcombe, & Riederle, 1993) suggests that sexual problems may be a primary symptom of severe or chronic sexual abuse (Jehu & Gazan, 1983).

Sexual abuse may also produce somatic concerns or preoccupation when bodily vulnerability or a specific bodily site or function becomes associated with violation (Briere, 1992c). This somatization dynamic has been associated with post–sexual-abuse trauma in several studies (Briere & Runtz, 1988; Drossman, Leserman, Nachman, Li, Gluck, Toomey, & Mitchel, 1990; Morrison, 1989; Springs & Friedrich, 1992) and is thought to underlie the specific reports of chronic pelvic pain in some female abuse survivors (Haber & Roos, 1985; Gross, Doerr, Caldirola, Guzinski, & Ripley, 1980–81; Walker, Katon, Harrop-Griffiths, Holm, Russo, & Hickok, 1988).

As noted earlier, these various manifestations of anxiety arise, to some degree, from the physical trauma and powerlessness that accompany (and become conditioned to) childhood sexual abuse. As well, it is likely that the child's early and continuous awareness of danger precludes the formation of a belief in a safe, just world—eventually leading to an adolescent or adult who understands the world to be a dangerous place where constant vigilance and a defensive stance are imperative for continued survival.

As a probable result of these factors, several DSM-IV anxiety disorders are overrepresented among adult sexual abuse survivors, as well as victims of other forms of child abuse—above and beyond those who satisfy criteria for PTSD (Saunders, et al., 1992; Stein, Golding, Siegel, Burnham, & Sorenson, 1988).

Depression

DSM-IV describes depression as sad mood "or loss of interest or pleasure in all or almost all activities" (p. 320) and lists the following symptoms as common: poor appetite, sleep disturbance, psychomotor retardation or agitation, loss of interest or pleasure in usual activities, decreased sex drive, loss of energy, feelings of worthlessness, self-reproach, excessive or inappropriate guilt, impaired concentration, recurrent thoughts about death, suicidal ideation, wishes to be dead, and suicide attempts. It further discriminates between "major depressive disorder," which involves a relatively intense and circumscribed period where these symptoms are present, and "dysthymic disorder," a milder form that typically has a longer course.

Theories of the etiology of depression stress a variety of factors, most of which are directly relevant to the experience of sexual abuse victims. These include early loss and abandonment (Bowlby, 1973); rejecting, punitive, and uncaring parent–child relationships (Blatt, Wein, Chevron, & Quinlan, 1979); chronic negative, self-blaming cognitions developed during childhood (Beck, 1967); and "learned helplessness" arising from chronic experiences of having no control over painful or aversive events (Seligman, 1975). Given the importance of these factors, and the frequency of such experiences in the lives of sexual abuse victims, we might reasonably predict that "in the clinical literature, depression is the symptom most commonly reported among adults molested as children" (Browne & Finkelhor, 1986a, p. 152).

The research literature highlights the frequency of depressive episodes among sexual abuse survivors as well. The National Institute of Mental Health–Los Angeles Catchment Area Study (Stein et al., 1988) reported that sexually abused women in the general population had almost a 4 times greater risk of developing a major depression than did women without such a history. Bagley and Ramsay (1986) found that in a community sample of 387 women, those with a history of childhood sexual abuse were approximately twice as likely to be clinically depressed as were women with no history of sexual abuse. Similarly, Peters (1984) found that a random community sample of women who had experienced sexually abusive contact as a child had an average of 2 times more depressive episodes in their lives than nonabused women and were more likely to have been hospitalized for depression. Other studies that have examined the relationship between childhood sexual abuse and depressive symptoms have typically found this connection (Briere & Runtz, 1987; Jehu, Gazan, & Klassen, 1984–85; Lipovsky, Saunders, & Murphy, 1989; Runtz, 1987; Saunders et al., 1992). This tendency toward depression may also explain partially the higher incidence of suicidal ideation and suicide attempts in sexual abuse survivors. Several studies have found that suicide attempts are more than 2 times more likely among mental health clients with sexual abuse histories than those without (Briere & Runtz, 1986; Briere & Zaidi, 1989; Herman, 1981; Sedney & Brooks, 1984).

In her discussion of the clinical presentation of sexual abuse survivors, Gelinas (1981) notes that

> most incest victims will not request treatment for incest, but for symptoms relating to longstanding depressions. The criteria for Dysthymic Disorders in the [DSM-III] provides a good characterization of this type of depression. However, incest victims show atypical depression with strong dissociative and impulsive elements. (p. 488)

Gelinas specifically refers to a sort of "needy depressiveness," which includes a mixture of anxious, depressive, and self/interpersonal symptomatology. In a similar vein, Briere and Runtz (1987) suggest that the clinical picture presented by the symptomatic sexual abuse survivor is often an amalgam of many types of symptoms such that a variety of DSM labels, including Major Depression or Dysthymic Disorder, are often applied.

Anger

Childhood sexual abuse can produce chronic irritability, unexpected or uncontrollable feelings of anger, and difficulties associated with the expression of anger in both child victims (Everson, Huner, & Rayan, 1991; Friedrich, Beilke, Urquiza, 1988; Lanktree, Briere, & Zaidi, 1991; Reich & Gutierres, 1979) and adult survivors (Bagley, 1991; Briere & Runtz, 1987; Briere et al., 1995; Donaldson & Gardner, 1985; Lipovsky et al., 1989). Because intense anger is a largely unacceptable affect in our culture, its expression is often suppressed or misdirected. This cultural prohibition against feeling, let alone expressing, intense or prolonged anger is likely to be especially unhelpful for the abuse survivor for several reasons. First, more sexual abuse survivors are women than men, and women have traditionally been judged more harshly than men when they express anger or hostility. Second, the survivor often has more legitimate reasons to be angry than many others, given the extent of maltreatment and injustice associated with her or his abuse. Third, the survivor's anger was often driven underground at the time of the abuse by virtue of fear of the perpetrator, causing him or her especially to acquiesce to social sanctions against angry expressions. Lastly, based on social, perpetrator, or family reactions to his appropriate rage, the survivor may have come to see his (unwanted but unavoidable) anger as evidence of abuse-related badness or psychopathology.

The suppression or misdirection of anger in abuse survivors can be quite detrimental. In the former case, angry feelings can become internalized as self-hatred and depression, occasionally providing the motive force for especially injurious instances of self-harm. A common clinical scenario, for example, is the survivor whose rage at herself (for, from her perspective, being so bad, stupid, ugly, or sluttish that others abused her) leads to self-mutilation involving deep and especially painful cuts or extended burns, suicide attempts involving especially painful methods (e.g., drinking Drano or stabbing herself in the abdomen), or especially humiliating or degrading "acting out," such as sexual contact with unusually unappealing or abusive individuals.

Socially and psychologically unacceptable anger may also be externalized by the survivor, sometimes resulting in the perpetration of abuse against others (Briere & Smiljanich, 1993; Carmen, Reiker, & Mills, 1984; Stukas-Davis, 1990) or other aggressive acts. The fact that certain especially violent or exploitive acts can be traced back to a childhood history of (sometimes equally abhorrent) victimization has led to a quandary for those concerned with abuse survivors. On one hand, the violent acts of a minority of abuse survivors are—in some sense—symptoms of abuse, in the same way as can be posttraumatic stress or depression. Conversely, the recent use of "abuse excuse" defenses by trial lawyers has both diminished the need to hold people responsible for their acts and has fed the public backlash against survivors (Briere, 1995a).

Although the resolution of this "symptom versus responsibility" dilemma (in some ways a recapitulation of the age-old philosophical problem of free will vs. determinism) far exceeds the grasp of this book, it may helpful to see abuse as an event that, for some individuals, increases the likelihood of—but in no way guarantees—aggressive behavior. For such individuals, involvement in violent or injurious acts against others may be a way to externalize or expel through action chronic rageful states. To the extent that such behaviors are within the survivor's conscious control, however, they remain chosen acts for which the survivor must take legal and psychological responsibility. However, when they are not under the survivor's control they should not be judged as such—as would be true of other, non–abuse-related instances of diminished capacity or irresistible impulse.

INTERPERSONAL EFFECTS

Because child abuse occurs, by definition, within the context of some sort of relationship, however brief or destructive, sexual abuse survivors often experience problems in the interpersonal domain. As noted by Berliner and Wheeler (1987): "From their abuse children learn certain patterns of behavior that are harmful to themselves or others, or that restrict their development and prevent them from attaining adequate functioning" (p. 420). Such effects are often very painful to the survivor, since they are associated with feelings of alienation, believing oneself to be incapable of having a "normal" (i.e., satisfying and relatively less conflictual) relationship, and a sometimes chronic and dysphoric neediness associated with early attachment-related difficulties. In addition, the survivor's childhood experience may produce generalized feelings of anger and rage, mixed with fearfulness—emotions easily evoked in later interactions with others. Despite their frequently negative impact, the interpersonal sequelae of sexual abuse may be understood as, in part, necessary accommodations the child was forced to make to survive the abuse process (Summit, 1983).

Clinicians have reported a variety of sexual-abuse–related difficulties in the interpersonal area, most of which have been further documented in the empirical literature. These may best be understood in terms of two general and overlapping groups of problems: (a) disturbed relatedness, and (b) "acting out" and "acting in."

Disturbed Relatedness

Sexual abuse may be relatively unique among forms of interpersonal aggression in that it combines exploitation and invasion with, in some instances, what might otherwise be evidence of love or caring (e.g., physical contact, cuddling, praise, and perhaps some positive physical sensations). As Butler notes: "Such activity is not always traumatic and frightening at the time it occurs if the father is not physically abusive, because he is able to count on his daughter's inability to understand the inappropriateness of his behavior and the warmth and sensual feelings his fondling generates in her" (1978, p. 32). To some extent this mixture may even be found in sexual abuse where "loving" was not present (e.g., where the abuse was more obviously forced) because in a general context of physical or emotional maltreatment or neglect, any attention or validation (if only for one's sexual value) may be perceived as positive. Further, as noted by Jill Blake-White and Christine Kline (1985):

> The fact that the perpetrator is a trusted adult makes her ambivalent and confused by her own feelings, and she may even doubt her own reality. She wonders if she had experienced a punishment or if she had elicited the incest by her own sexuality. (p. 396)

Given this concatenation of stimuli, many sexual abuse survivors are highly ambivalent about intimate relationships—especially ones where sexual or romantic themes predominate.

Idealization and Disappointment

Such ambivalence may express itself as mixed and sometimes contradictory motivations for relating to others. Thus, survivors may feel distrust or fear of others in combination with a paradoxical tendency to idolize individuals they perceive or want to perceive as "good." Herman (1981), for example, found in her sample of female abuse victims that "the majority of the incest victims, in fact, tended to overvalue and idealize men" (p. 103). As upcoming chapters on psychotherapy and "borderline dynamics" indicate, such idealization often leads to disappointment and anger, both because of the survivor's underlying distrust and rage, which may stimulate less than ideal responses from others, and the tendency for the idolized to inevitably emerge as human at some point. Thus, an unfortunate effect of the idealization process can be frequent, intense, but highly unstable attachments to others that end in anger and further loss.

> Peggy is a 34-year-old woman lives alone in an apartment with her two cats. She seeks therapy "to become more of a woman." Although a bit of a loner at work, she frequents singles bars at night in search of "male companionship." At the end of these forays. Peggy frequently brings a man home with her but rarely hears from him again after that night. She describes most of these men positively, and she bitterly speculates about what it is about her that they just "do their number and leave." Further exploration reveals that she has been raped by two of these men and beaten by two others—events for which Peggy blames herself, citing her many negative qualities and shortcomings. She reports, on questioning, sexual abuse by an uncle and a friend of the family during most of her adolescence.

Another result of the idealization dynamic can be *revictimization*. This term refers to the findings of several studies (Elliott & Mok, 1995; Fromuth, 1985; McCord, 1985; Runtz, 1987; Russell, 1986; Woo & Briere, 1992) that female sexual abuse survivors are more likely to be victimized again later in life (e.g., via rape or battering) than are women with no history of childhood sexual abuse. Although several explanations have been offered for this phenomenon, one possibility is that in their drive to see men in a positive light, some survivors may overlook cues or behaviors that nonabused women would see as danger signs, such as aggressiveness or extreme authoritarianism. Further, when confronted with abusive behavior, the survivor may be more prone to "forgive and forget"; both because she learned long ago to avoid contact with threatening stimuli and in the hope that her current abuser will redeem himself in ways that her original perpetrator(s) did not.

Given the complexity of this phenomenon and the potential for such behavior to be erroneously labeled as masochistic (Runtz & Briere, 1988) or for the victim to be seen as deserving her abuse, further research is clearly indicated in this area. Additional reasons for revictimization may include that (a) the survivor's low self-esteem may lead her to assume that abusive individuals are all that she deserves (Conte & Schuerman (1987; Courtois, 1988), (b) the learned helplessness arising from sexual abuse may create victims who become passive in the face of impending victimization (McCord, 1985), (c) abusive men may learn to identify women who have been previously abused and thus are easy prey, and (d) the frequently impaired self-functions of the severely abused survivor may result in a decreased ability to detect boundary violations or to reject the persuasiveness of the sexual victimizer (Briere, 1992a).

Intimacy Problems or Sexualized Relatedness

A dynamic similar to that of idealization is sometimes present in the abuse survivor's sexual relationships. On the one hand, she has seen for herself the potential for sex to include exploitation and trauma, and thus appropriately fears the vulnerability and intimacy inherent in sexual relationships. This fear may lead not only to sexual dysfunction and powerful dissociative states during sexual contact, but also to a general distrust of sex partners and men in general (Courtois, 1988; Jehu, Gazan, & Klassen, 1984–85; Maltz, 1988; Meiselman, 1978), and generic difficulties with intimacy (Courtois, 1988; Elliott, 1994). Yet as described by Herman (1981): "At the same time that these women had little hope of attaining a rewarding relationship with anyone, they desperately longed for the nurturance and care which they had not received in childhood" (p. 100).

Having learned at an early age that one of their most powerful assets in gaining some sort of contact with or control over others was their sexual availability, many sexual abuse survivors report periods of compulsive or dysfunctional sexual behavior (Briere et al., 1995; Briere & Runtz, 1990b; Courtois, 1979a; Herman, 1981; Meiselman, 1978). The frequent yet short-lived nature of these sexual encounters can thus be understood as the need to seek nurturance, love, power, and self-affirmation in the only way thought possible, while, at the same time, addressing historically valid fears of exploitation and only partially suppressed rage at having been so deeply hurt by "similar" individuals. This complex dynamic may become a vicious cycle for some women, wherein the survivor (a) behaves in a flirtatious or seductive manner with those from whom she seeks approval or rescue from emptiness and isolation, which (b) places her at risk from predatory individuals who frequently exploit and victimize her, motivating (c) her increasing sense of aloneness and belief that "all men (or women) are alike" in terms of their needs or perceptions, thereby (d) further verifying to the survivor that her only value with regard to others is the transient attraction of her sex.

The stereotypic male version of this dynamic is somewhat less complex, although equally painful for the survivor and those around him. The survivor may (a) seek out sexual contact as a way to gain nurturance, support, and validation; (b) find such superficial contact unsatisfying after the initial excitement has faded and the person involved appears to make excessive demands (e.g., for intimacy or relationship); leading to (c) a search for new, "better" partners.

Along with the use of sexuality (narrowly described) for its impacts on others, survivors may engage in frequent sexual activity to address painful internal states. The extremity of the survivor's abuse-related distress may lead him to use sexual contact as a way to soothe painful feelings, distract himself from intrusive memories and affects, elicit positive responses from others (thereby neutralizing some of his own self-derogation), fill perceived emptiness, and provide distress-incompatible stimulation. Unfortunately, like other *tension-reduction* activities (see chapter 3 for more on this concept), such behavior typically is effective in the short-term only, leading to more seemingly compulsive or "addictive" sexual behavior in the future.

Adversariality

Although some survivors of severe sexual abuse may be ambivalent regarding to their contacts with others, they are often clearer, as noted earlier, about how to engage in such interactions. They often learned during childhood that things are gained primarily through exchange of other things—never inherently deserved and thus never freely given. This adversarial perspective assumes that love, caring, physical goods, or attention are available to only the survivor if she trades sex for them or tricks someone into providing them. The former, which we shall refer to as *sexual adversariality*, is commonly seen in adolescent street kids and teenage prostitutes, whose cynicism about their ultimate value to others may be startling.

Various studies have documented an association between sexual abuse and subsequent teenage prostitution, noting that 60% to 73% of three groups of adolescent prostitutes were sexually abused as children (Bagley & Young, 1987; James & Meyerding, 1977; Silbert & Pines, 1981). In fact, prostitution is described by some survivors as one of the most representative of human interactions because it involves the exchange of sex for money, just as the (forced) exchange in childhood was for attention, validation, or escape from injury.

Such adversariality is not limited to overtly sexual actions, however. The survivor may also service her therapist with compliments, flirtations, superficial agreement, and "good client" behaviors to ensure continuing therapeutic contact and support, or may tolerate abusive behavior from a spouse, partner, or employer to ensure continued security or to forestall abandonment.

Finally, this adversarial perspective often manifests as a chronic tendency to view interpersonal interactions as battles, which the former child abuse victim seeks to win (or lose) to survive. Given his childhood experience of injustice (i.e., the unfairness of being hurt but not rescued, and of the abuser being bad but not punished), he may decide early in life that "all bets are off" regarding cultural notions of honesty or fairness. In the vacuum that this perception creates, the survivor may learn to use almost any options he has available to him to prevail in his interactions with others. This survival pattern can motivate one of the behaviors most often attributed by clinicians to borderline personality disorder—that of manipulation.

Manipulation

As typically understood, manipulation refers to those behaviors engaged in by an individual to receive goods or services from others who would not otherwise bestow them. As is noted in an upcoming section, this behavior is especially worrisome to some psychotherapists, who may fear that they are being taken advantage of or exploited in some way. From the victim's perspective, however, manipulativeness can be seen as a historically appropriate survival behavior. Such actions appear to be based on several underlying dynamics: (a) low self-esteem, (b) the survivor's belief that nothing good is freely given, and (c) his or her previously developed skills at extracting needed resources from a hostile environment (i.e., "survival" per se).

Although, from the former sexual abuse victim's perspective, the intent of adversarial behaviors is survival, a typical result is social isolation and rejection—especially when the ambivalent dynamics of rage, neediness, and distrust are present. Specifically, the sexual abuse survivor's difficulties in relating to others can result in a tendency to withdraw from the social milieu or to be rejected by it.

These feelings, often exacerbated by coexisting depression, may make it especially difficult for the survivor to reach out for help or support from others, thereby potentially increasing his or her sense of isolation. Alternatively, this alienation may produce increased emotional neediness, leading to inappropriate interpersonal behaviors (as described in the next section), and, as a result, subsequent greater rejection and estrangement.

Acting-Out versus Adaptive or Functional Behavior

Several writers have noted that adolescents and adults who were severely abused as children are prone to a variety of socially problematic behaviors. Such behavior is often referred to as "acting out," a term commonly used to describe acts that are self-destructive or harmful to others, and that are thought to arise from internal conflict. In the case of child abuse, such behaviors include truancy and other school problems (Reich & Gutierres, 1979; Runtz & Briere, 1986), running away from home (McCormack, Janus, & Burgess, 1986), aggression (Bagley, 1984; Reich & Gutierres, 1979), drug and alcohol abuse (Briere & Zaidi, 1989; Dembo et al., 1989; Miller, Downs, Gondoli, & Keil, 1987), self-mutilation (van der Kolk, Perry, & Herman, 1991; Walsh & Rosen, 1988), delinquency or criminality (Pollock, Briere, Schneider, Knop, Mednick, & Goodwin, 1990; Ross, 1980), and those behaviors described in earlier sections—prostitution, suicidality and "promiscuity."

A casual review of these behaviors reveals their heterogeneity, with the only obvious common quality being their tendency to be seen as trouble by others—perhaps especially by caregivers and law enforcers. Such behaviors arise from a variety of motivations or underlying psychological processes, as opposed to some hypothetical unitary quality reflecting "adjustment problems" or "borderline" behaviors. At minimum, however, we may understand these different behaviors as abuse-specific instrumental responses, frequently involving avoidance activities and tension-reduction behaviors. However, rarely will these behaviors be described as "self-destructive" in this book because this term implies that such activities represent the survivor's attempts to punish or even destroy herself in response to abuse-related self-hatred. Although some survivors' self-hatred may be so severe that self-destruction is sought, most other so-called self-destructive behaviors are, in reality, survival activities. The very notion of a self-destructive survivor, in fact, is an oxymoron.

Abuse-related instrumental behaviors are those activities that were adaptive during the period in which sexual abuse occurred, but that may or may not be relevant to the postabuse environment. Behaviors seemingly maladaptive in the current context may be continued because, as described in the Cognitive Effects section, sexual victimization frequently distorts subsequent perceptions of the self and the world, producing behaviors that are situationally, but not historically, inappropriate. For example, the survivor's view of herself as bad, unworthy, and unlovable, in combination with a perception of others as untrustworthy and the world as dangerous, may support what appears to be needless attention getting, manipulativeness, or delinquency. Other behaviors, such as stereotypically seductive behavior, may be continued based on the survivor's belief that her only asset as an adult is her stimulus value to others, and the acts she can perform or the compliance she can offer.

Other supposed "acting out" behaviors can be adaptive in the postabuse environment, albeit typically in only the short term. As noted by writers, such as Reich and Gutierres (1979) and Lindberg and Distad (1985b), for example, certain behaviors (e.g., substance abuse) may allow the survivor to avoid distressing external situations. Other behaviors (e.g., self-mutilation or "compulsive" sexual behavior) may reduce painful internal states or tension, as indicated earlier. Finally, some survivor behaviors may represent attempts to communicate through action messages that, for whatever reason, cannot be spoken directly.

Drug and alcohol abuse appear to serve as a form of chemically induced dissociation for some survivors, allowing him or her to escape from abuse-related memories or painful mood states. The frequency of this avoidance defense is suggested by the findings of one study that psychotherapy clients with a history of sexual abuse are more than twice as likely to have a history of alcoholism and 10 times more likely to report having been addicted to drugs in the past than a control group of nonabused clients (Briere & Runtz, 1987). This numbing or mood-altering effect of drugs and alcohol is so substantial that psychotherapy is often considerably less effective when the survivor is regularly using such substances.

Self-mutilation is an especially good example of the adaptive and yet ultimately self-injurious nature of certain tension-reduction behaviors (Gil & Briere, 1995; Walsh & Rosen, 1988). Intentional yet nonsuicidal self-injury (e.g., cutting or carving on one's arms or legs, or burning oneself with matches or cigarettes) is sometimes described by survivors as an effective way to

- Terminate dissociative episodes. In the words of one survivor: "I had done it because I was feeling scared that I was beginning not to feel anything. I needed to see if I was still real, if I could still hurt" (Butler, 1978, p. 45).

- Distract themselves from painful memories or flashbacks (what one survivor described as "using new pain to hide old pain").
- Communicate to others the presence of internal (invisible) pain by making external (visible) wounds.
- Provide relief from guilt, by way of self-punishment.
- Reassure themselves that they are alive and "in reality."
- Increase their sense of autonomy. As one male survivor put it: "I can do whatever I want to my body. When I hurt myself, it is me doing it and me feeling it."

As would be predicted by a tension-reduction perspective, survivors who self-mutilate often describe a period of escalating guilt, self-disgust, and self-criticism just before self-injury. After the act, these negative cognitions usually abate, and a period of calm and almost palpable relief may ensue (Gil & Briere, 1995). Unfortunately for the chronic self-mutilator, this pattern is likely to recur in the near future with the onset of "new" (in actuality, typically old but unresolved) guilt or self-derogating cognitions.

As described earlier, Alice was brought to the emergency room of a local hospital during a severe dissociative episode. After being admitted to a psychiatric unit, numerous old and recent scars were found on her abdomen, thighs, arms, and wrists during a routine physical examination. Alice admits that these healed and healing wounds are due to intentional self-injury, primarily involving lacerations with razor blades, but also including what appear to be cigarette burns. Records from a previous hospitalization indicate that, on one occasion, Alice cut an 8-inch opening in her inner thigh, which extended nearly to the bone.

In contrast to the seemingly compulsive quality of repetitive self-mutilation, survivors with suicidal ideation may report an ongoing preoccupation with dying and death, usually as a result of feelings of helplessness and hopelessness, and a combination of anger at self (for being so weak/disgusting/stupid/etc.) and others (for not caring/loving/supporting/etc.). These suicidal thoughts and impulses are typically chronic, often dating back to the time of the original sexual abuse. Briere and Runtz (1986) for example, found that of 14 women who had made a suicide attempt before age 13, 13 (93%) reported having been sexually abused.

Suicidal behavior often represents an extreme form of avoidance. Suicidal survivors in treatment frequently note that their desire is not to approach death but rather to avoid the overwhelming emotional pain of life. In other words, for such individuals, death provides the ultimate dissociation from overwhelming psychic pain, as opposed to being a state worth approaching in its own right.

Intentionally nonlethal suicidal behavior (so-called suicidal gestures) also may represent a cry for help in individuals who believe that they have no other effective way of communicating psychological pain. Thus, suicidal behaviors in some abuse survivors may reflect the belief that extraordinary measures are required to gain the caring attention of others, given their perceived lack of power and undeservingness in more conventional contexts.

The ultimate motives for self-mutilation and suicide are often notably different, despite the tendency for some writers and clinicians (including the authors of DSM-III-R and DSM-IV) to see them as similar reflections of self-destructiveness. In many cases, the self-mutilator is struggling to stay alive, using external methods to modulate overwhelmingly painful internal states, whereas the suicidal survivor is considering death. For example, one study of people diagnosed with borderline personality disorder found that self-mutilatory behavior was *negatively* associated with suicidal behavior (McGlashan, 1986, cited in Krol, 1993, p. 27).

As mentioned earlier, self-mutilation is often an attempt to block or interrupt negative cognitions or feelings (e.g., dissociation, rage, extreme dysphoria, or overwhelming guilt) and thus may be an attempt to survive incapacitating symptoms rather than ending life. Even in cases where self-mutilation serves as self-punishment, it is often described by survivors as a substitute for more lethal behaviors (Gil & Briere, 1995). Thus, self-mutilation can—in some instances—be a sign of continuing struggle for symptom relief and survival, and, therefore, may be dealt with differently from intentionally self-lethal behaviors. It is important to note, however, that some intensely suicidal individuals (who may or may not be abuse survivors) also self-mutilate, sometimes describing the superficial slashing of wrists or the throat as "dry runs" before "the real thing." For this reason, self-mutilatory behavior should be assessed carefully for its function and meaning to the survivor before diagnostic or prognostic assumptions are made.

Summary

Taken together, the empirical and clinical literatures on the long-term effect of childhood sexual abuse provide little doubt that such victimization can be harmful and long lasting for many individuals. As opposed to other subjects in the behavioral sciences, the relationship between abuse and effects appears straightforward: Sexually abusive acts often hurt children and, in the absence of appropriate treatment, hurt children often grow to become hurt adults. The extent of this injury appears to be a function of many variables, including type, duration, and frequency of abuse; interpersonal resources available to the victim; who the offender was (i.e., father, brother, or teacher); when it occurred; how significant others responded to the abuse disclosure; and whether physical force was involved (see Berliner & Elliott [1996] and Browne & Finkelhor [1986a] for a review of the literature in this area). Despite the complexity of such mediating variables, however, few studies performed in the last 10 years show any form of childhood sexual abuse to be benign or harmless.

Why then, we might ask, has relatively little of this research penetrated into the basic clinical literature? If sexual abuse has been associated with anxiety, depression, dissociation, chemical dependency, self-injurious behavior, even personality disorders, why do the standard clinical texts on these subjects typically fail to mention sexual victimization and other forms of child abuse as potentially important etiological factors? Although answers to such questions are likely to include society's drive to deny the extent and implications of sexual victimization (as described in chapter 3), part of the problem appears to reside in the fact that clinicians *already* have explanations for many of these patterns without specific reference to sexual abuse. Thus, this blind spot is due not only to the relative newness of our information on sexual victimization (as opposed to the many years of theorizing entailed in extant theories of psychopathology) but also reflects the specific tendency of traditional theorists to discount abuse reports as fantasies. This disbelief is not limited to the days of yore, however, as witness contemporary media response to the "repressed memory" controversy.

As an example of the psychiatric redefinition of post–sexual-abuse trauma, and because of their special relevance to many survivors in the traditional psychiatric care system, the next chapter considers two commonly diagnosed mental disorders: Hysteria and borderline personality disorder. Chapter 2 also examines the nonpsychiatric label of *false memory syndrome* as it relates to both traditional psychiatric thinking and current social dynamics.

Hysteria, Borderline Personality Disorder, and False Memory Syndrome

2

Traditional theories of psychopathology often act to impede the clinicians' understanding of the relationship between child sexual abuse and a given client's psychological state. Because earlier theories often provide plausible—albeit potentially inaccurate—reasons for the client's behavior or complaints, more accurate information regarding the role of abuse trauma may be dismissed by the therapist who believes he already possesses a valid explanation. This explanation typically is accompanied by a psychiatric diagnosis, which, in turn, may become a self-fulfilling prophesy regarding subsequent interpretations of the survivor's behavior.

Perhaps the two most common diagnoses applied to survivors of severe childhood sexual abuse are hysteria (or histrionic personality disorder) and borderline personality disorder. Each diagnosis is thought to have some descriptive utility in that, for example, most clinicians believe they know more about a person once she or he is described as "borderline" or "histrionic" than they did before. Unfortunately, however, the assumptions they immediately make about the person—in terms of presenting difficulties, etiology, treatment, and prognosis—may not be entirely accurate, perhaps especially when the client has a history of severe sexual abuse.

Hysteria

As described in one psychiatric dictionary (Campbell, 1989), hysteria refers to a constellation of symptoms including (a) physical problems for which no organic cause can be found (e.g., paralysis, tics, or tremors); (b) alterations in sensation (e.g., loss of feeling in areas of the body, persistent tingling, or sudden blindness); (c) "visceral" symptoms (e.g., "anorexia, bulimia, vomiting, hiccup[s] . . . [and] various abdominal complaints"); and (d) "mental" symptoms, including amnesia, somnambulism (sleepwalking), and "fugues, trances, dream states, [and] hysterical fits or attacks" (p. 344).

Although hysteria is no longer an accepted diagnosis in current psychiatric nomenclature (i.e., in DSM-IV), it remains a common explanation among mental health clinicians for the behavior of (almost always) women whose physical or psychological complaints appear groundless or overstated. A related diagnosis, that of Histrionic Personality Disorder, however, remains in DSM-IV. Campbell (1989) describes this disorder as including

> any or all of the following: vain, egocentric, attention-seeking, dramatic descriptions of past symptoms and illnesses with a multiplicity of vaguely described complaints and overtalkativeness during the psychiatric interview; suggestibility; soft, coquettish, graceful, and sexually provocative although frigid and anxious when close to attaining a sexual goal; easily disappointed, excitable, emotionally labile, and often unaware of inner feelings; dependently demanding in interpersonal situations. . . . Such a manipulative adaptational pattern occurs in those with a tendency toward rigid repression of dysphoric emotion. . . . Conflicts in such patients are often centered around *genital incest strivings,* [emphasis added] and/or oral disappointments." (p. 369)

To this list DSM-IV adds: discomfort in situations where he or she is not the center of attention, inappropriate sexually seductive or provocative behavior, rapidly shifting and shallow emotional expression, use of physical appearance to call attention to self, impressionistic speech, self-dramatization, hypersuggestibility, and assumption of more intimacy in relationships than actually exists (pp. 657–658).

The reader will no doubt recognize many of these responses as having been linked (it is hoped in a less pejorative manner) to childhood sexual victimization in the literature cited in chapter 1. Among other symptoms, hysteria and severe post–sexual-abuse trauma appear to share (a) dissociation in its various forms, (b) somatic complaints, (c) problems with sexuality, (d) problems with affect tolerance and regulation, and (e) a variety of interpersonal difficulties (e.g., ambivalence, idealization, attention getting, sexualization, dependency, and manipulation). Briere and Runtz (1987, 1988a) specifically document similar abuse-related symptoms (dissociation, dysphoria, somatization, and interpersonal dysfunction) in both clinical and nonclinical samples of sexual abuse survivors, whereas Herman (1986) and Rosenfeld (1979) found similar clusters of "hysterical" symptoms in abuse survivors within two psychiatric outpatient samples. As Herman eloquently notes, "the hysteric, although banished from DSM-III, is still frequently seen as a psychiatric patient, and she is still suffering, as Freud noted long ago, from memories" (p. 13).

> Emilia is a bright, intense 22-year-old woman entered a therapy group for "adult children of alcoholics" at a local community center. Initially liked by most group members for her wit, charm, and seeming openness, she gradually becomes ostracized from the group—partially as a result of her sexual involvement with two older group members, who subsequently stop coming to meetings. It becomes clear as well that Emilia needs to be the center of the group's attention, and she becomes increasingly angry and depressed as the group begins to ignore her. With the passage of time, Emilia's superficially cheerful and excited facade disappears, and her underlying loneliness and poor self-esteem become obvious. During session number eight, Emilia reveals that her alcoholic father sexually molested her from ages 7 to 16, and still approaches her at family reunions. She tearfully relates times when her father would call her "my little baby" as he penetrated her sexually.

Other writers have also described specific "hysterical" symptoms in victims of sexual abuse, including several reports of hysterical seizures or pseudoepilepsy (Goodwin, Simms, & Bergman, 1979; Gross, 1979; McAnarney, 1975). A typical case history (one of four) was presented by Goodwin et al. (1979):

A. was . . . hospitalized at age 14 following convulsions in the deten-
tion center in which she was placed after running away from home
for the second time. Two weeks previously, her natural father had
intercourse with her. . . . She said her father had been seductive with
her before, as had a maternal uncle. The father admitted having had
intercourse with her. A. was sexually active with peers and had
threatened suicide. She said that she was conscious during the
seizures and that they usually occurred when she was alone. . . . Elec-
troencephalogram was normal. Conversion disorder with hysterical
seizures was diagnosed. Psychotherapy was begun and the seizures
disappeared, but promiscuity and runaways continued as problems.
(p. 699)

Although concurring with the presence of certain "hysterical"
symptoms in some sexual abuse survivors, the findings of the sexual abuse literature would not be in concordance with the notion
that such individuals are struggling with "genital incest strivings"
as described by Campbell (1989, p. 346). The history of how trauma
arising from sexual victimization could be redefined as the results
of the survivor's childhood striving for incest may appear bizarre
to those not familiar with the Freudian model of psychosexual
development. Although the basic outlines of this phenomenon will
be briefly described here, the reader is referred to Hannah Lerman's
(1986) *A Mote in Freud's Eye: From Psychoanalysis to the Psychology of
Women* and Jeffrey Masson's (1984) *The Assault on Truth: Freud's Suppression of the Seduction Theory.*

Freud's View of Hysteria and the "Oedipal Complex"

As Campbell (1989) notes, Freud's initial work with his female
patients led him to believe that

the hysterical attack was a symbolic representation of a repressed sexual trauma. He believed that the patient had undergone a passive sexual experience in childhood, but that this psychical experience could
not find adequate discharge because the nervous system was incapable of dealing with it at that time; the experience was forgotten, but
with puberty the memory of it was reawakened. . . . This theory was
later revised [by Freud] *when it was discovered that the sexual traumata*

> *uncovered in hysterical patients were really fictitious memories designed to*
> *mask the autoerotic activities of childhood* [emphasis added]. (p. 344)

In Freud's own words,

> Almost all my women patients told me that they had been seduced
> by their fathers. I was driven to recognize in the end that these reports
> were untrue and so came to understand that the hysterical symptoms
> are derived from phantasies and not from real occurrences. . . . It was
> only later that I was able to recognize in this phantasy of being
> seduced by the father the expression of the typical Oedipus complex
> in women. (cited in Rush, 1980, p. 83)

In a similar vein, Freud concluded in *The Interpretation of Dreams*
(1900) that "the theory of the psychoneurosis asserts as an indis-
putable and invariable fact that only sexual wishful impulses from
infancy, which have undergone repression . . . are able to furnish the
motive force for the formation of psychoneurotic symptoms"
(pp. 605–606). As Judith Herman (1981) notes in *Father-Daughter
Incest*, Freud's sudden change of heart regarding the basis for his
clients' incest reports "was based not on any new evidence from
patients [i.e., the "discoveries" reported by Campbell], but rather on
Freud's own growing unwillingness to believe that licentious behavior on the part of fathers could be so widespread" (p. 10).

Freud's concerns about the implications of his original theory for
the frequency of incest in his culture are reproduced at length by
Masson (1984), who quotes from Freud's letters to his friend and col-
league Wilhelm Fleiss. Among other misgivings, Freud states that
"surely such widespread perversions against children are not very
probable" (p. 108). As was noted in the introduction to this book,
current data suggest that incest and sexual abuse are relatively common in our society and indicate that, in fact, the (especially female)
caseloads of many clinicians do contain a significant number of sexual abuse survivors—data to which Freud, of course, had no access.

Freud's ultimate belief, his theory of the Oedipus complex, was
that boys and girls sexually desired their opposite-sexed parent and,
through a complex series of events including male fear of castration
and female envy of penises, ultimately developed rich fantasies of

seducing said parent—fantasies that some could not differentiate from reality at later points in their lives (hence, the "hysterical" reports of incest). Freud further hypothesized that it was the *mother*, in fact, who was responsible for any childhood sexual stimulation. As cited by Lerman (1986, p. 105), Freud concluded in 1931 that

> this is because they [children] necessarily received their first, or at any rate their strongest, genital sensations when they were being cleaned and having their toilet attended to by their mothers. . . . The fact that the mother thus unavoidably initiates the child into the phallic phase is, I think, the reason why in phantasies of later years, the father so regularly appears as the sexual seducer. (p. 238)

Several writers (Enns et al., 1995; Herman, 1981; Lerman, 1986; Masson, 1984; Miller, 1984; Rush, 1980) seriously question both the empirical and logical basis for Freud's Oedipal theory of psychosexual development and discount his theory regarding the "fictitious" nature of his female clients' sexual abuse reports. In the words of Hannah Lerman (1986): "Freud's knowledge of female sexuality was limited, to put it most charitably. It was due to the sparse information available in his time. His theory, which is built on very scant and often erroneous evidence, nevertheless became quite expansive and authoritative" (p. 84).

Freud's theoretical misstep has had major implications for the future of mental health practice because it (a) introduced a probably false (but nevertheless immensely popular) set of assumptions regarding the etiology of "hysteria" and other psychological maladies and (b) set a precedent for following generations of psychotherapists to disbelieve their clients' (especially women's) reports of childhood sexual victimization.

It is not particularly useful or even intellectually honest, however, to blame writings from the first years of this century for what continues to be, in essence, a broadly social phenomenon. One may ask, for example, what other scientific discipline would continue to rely on relatively nonempirical theories developed nearly 100 years ago when attempting to address a major contemporary problem. Clearly, for such archaic theorizing to have such a long shelf life, it must address a continuing social need. This need, whether conscious or otherwise, seems to be to underestimate steadfastly the incidence and impacts of childhood sexual abuse, and to counter those who continue to raise the issue at a social level.

As a study of contemporary psychoanalytic writings will attest, the tendency to discount individuals who report incest or other sexual abuse continues in some circles—as does a reliance on some form of Oedipal interpretation. Although fewer authorities are willing to denounce a client's incest report as a total falsehood, there is often the strong implication or direct statement that Oedipal strivings caused the client to actively pursue her abuser, who was then unable to resist the temptation. From such a perspective, the clinician may reject the notion of the survivor as victim and thereby deny any injuries arising from the abuse. James Henderson, for example, noted two decades ago in the *Comprehensive Textbook of Psychiatry* (the major teaching reference in psychiatry) that

> the daughters collude in the incestuous liaison and play an active and even initiating role in establishing the pattern . . . [she] is unlikely to report the liaison at first or to protest about it. If she eventually does, it is as much precipitated by anger at her father for something else . . . as a real objection to his incestuous behavior. (1975, p. 1356)

What makes this phenomenon all the more unfortunate is that women who display "hysterical" symptoms in therapy and who also report sexual abuse are probably the most likely to be discounted, despite the possible cause-effect relationship between such symptoms and the sexual abuse. Her "sexually provocative," "coquettish," or "easily excitable" style may instead be interpreted as evidence of her prior collusion with her abuser, or her abuse disclosure may be seen as fiction in the service of arousing or seducing the therapist. As chapters 4 and 6 discuss, successful psychotherapy with the sexual abuse survivor demands a high level of respect and support for his or her experience, and an understanding acceptance of whatever survival behaviors he or she may need to display during therapy—a treatment approach that many survivors with previous therapy experiences find novel. Alice Miller, the Swiss psychoanalyst, notes this well when she states:

In every psychiatric and psychoanalytic diagnosis, the description of
a hysterical patient is inconceivable without the use of the word
"exaggerated." What is meant by this is that these patients' complaints are out of all proportion to their cause. But how can we measure the dimensions of the true cause if it is unknown or is ignored
by the therapist. (1984, pp 31–32)

Borderline Personality Disorder

Although the history of the concept of hysteria is inextricably
linked to Freud and his theory of feminine psychosexual development, the diagnosis of borderline personality disorder is a more
recent phenomenon. Probably because criteria for this diagnosis
include self-destructive behavior, identity disturbance, and relationship problems, it appears to be the most common psychiatric
label currently applied to survivors of severe sexual abuse.

DSM-IV describes borderline personality disorder—which it sees
as more common in women—as a chronic disturbance in which
there is "a pervasive pattern of instability of interpersonal relationship, self-image, and affects, and marked impulsivity beginning by
early adulthood and present in a variety of contexts" (American
Psychiatric Association, 1994, p. 650). The primary symptoms of borderline personality disorder, according to DSM IV are (1) "frantic
efforts to avoid real or imagined abandonment" (2) "a pattern of
unstable and intense interpersonal relationships" (e.g., idealization,
manipulation, and marked shifts in attitude), (3) "identity disturbance: markedly and persistently unstable self image or sense of
self," (4) "impulsivity in at least two areas that are potentially self
damaging," (e.g., spending, sex, substance use, reckless driving,
binge eating)," (5) "recurrent suicidal behavior, gestures, or threats,
or self-mutilating behavior," (6) "affective instability due to a
marked reactivity of mood," (7) "chronic feelings of emptiness," (8)
"inappropriate, intense anger or difficulty in controlling anger," and
(9) "transient, stress-related paranoid ideation or severe dissociative
symptoms" (p. 654).

The reader will note the close parallels between the preceding
and the pattern of problems seen in many adolescents and adults
who have experienced severe or prolonged sexual abuse in childhood. It can be shown, for example, that almost all of the symptoms

listed in the DSM-IV for borderline personality disorder have been independently reported as victimization effects in the sexual abuse literature. As a result, several studies (Briere & Zaidi, 1989; Fisher, 1991; Bryer, Nelson, Miller, & Krol, 1987; Herman, 1985; Herman, Perry, & van der Kolk, 1989; Lobel, 1990; Ogata et al., 1990), using widely disparate samples and diagnostic approaches, indicate that women with childhood histories of abuse may be considerably more likely than nonabused women to receive a diagnosis of borderline personality disorder. In addition, several writers (Briere, 1992a; Courtois, 1988; Gelinas, 1983; Herman & van der Kolk, 1987; Reiker & Carmen, 1986) suggest that early, sustained sexual abuse—perhaps especially in combination with early neglect-related attachment difficulties—predisposes some individuals to "borderline" behavior.

> Kathy is a 27-year-old woman who came to a university counseling center complaining of depression, emptiness, and continuing academic difficulties, the latter usually resulting in dropped classes and conflicts with professors. On intake interview, she described a long childhood history of sexual abuse by, initially, her father, followed by her stepfather when her father died. She reports an extensive history of suicide attempts, beginning at age 14 and continuing to her last attempt several months earlier. These suicide attempts often occur in the context of relationship difficulties and substance abuse, although she denies that drugs or alcohol are a problem. Kathy is quite engaging in the intake interview, and the intake clinician decides to include Kathy in her own caseload, despite the fact that her job is normally to distribute clients among the other counseling center therapists. After several sessions, however, Kathy starts to be seen as a "problem client," making repeated calls to the center, demanding multiple sessions a week, and eventually drawing several center personnel into her dealings with her therapist. She becomes increasingly angry at the therapist, claiming that she has abandoned the client by virtue of her limited availability. After several months of stormy interactions with the therapist, Kathy reveals deep cuts on both forearms, stating: "See what you made me do?"

Unfortunately, traditional mental health systems typically do not explain borderline symptomatology in terms of its possible relation to child abuse. As noted by Herman and van der Kolk (1987)

Occasional case examples that include severe physical or sexual abuse in the background of borderline patients are found throughout the literature; generally, they are reported without any comment on the possible impact of the trauma. In the main, the idea that borderline patients may in actuality have been severely abused tends to be discounted or dismissed as part of the patient's self-serving distortion of reality. (p. 114)

Instead of its potential connection to sexual abuse, this disturbance may be seen as resulting from "early object loss" and difficulties in the "separation-individuation" period of childhood. Interestingly, there has been considerable controversy in psychiatry over the specific symptoms of borderline personality disorder (see Gunderson & Singer [1975] and Perry & Klerman [1978] for reviews of the various features attributed to this syndrome). Despite this variability and given the steadying influence of concrete DSM-III and DSM-IV criteria, the diagnosis of borderline personality disorder has become increasingly frequent in inpatient and outpatient psychiatric settings.

Most theories of borderline development (Kernberg, 1975; Masterson, 1978) trace the genesis of this disorder to dysfunctional maternal behavior in the first year or two of the child's life. As a result of aversive mother-child interactions, the soon-to-be-borderline child is thought to be arrested at a pre-Oedipal level, such that she or he is unable to form the capacity for healthy object relations. According to one writer (Groves, 1975), "Whereas in normal development the child learns to separate from important objects [e.g., mother] with sadness and anger rather than with despair and rage, the borderline cannot tolerate negative affects associated with separation and continues into adulthood the pre-Oedipal child's clinging, as if others were desperately-needed parts rather than separate persons" (p. 338). A well-known analyst summarizes this process as follows:

> We have postulated that the mother of the future borderline child and adult, herself borderline, rewards (provides libidinal supplies and gratification to) her infant when he behaves in a dependent, clinging manner towards her, but threatens to reject or abandon . . . him when he makes efforts toward being independent of her, that is, toward sep-

aration-individuation. Thus, the infant (later the borderline individual) comes to perceive that independence, growth, and autonomy lead only to abandonment, while remaining symbiotically dependent guarantees the flow and acquisition of necessary support and supplies, albeit at the ultimate and disastrous expense of healthy independence and autonomy. Thus, the borderline individual's double bind; to remain infantile is to retain the mother and her love, to grow is to lose them (the ultimate meaning of the term loser). (Rinsley, 1980, p. 290)

The abuse perspective provided in this book is generally at odds with the preceding, given information that similar difficulties have been associated with severe child maltreatment, perhaps especially severe and early sexual abuse. Among other points of disagreement are the following:

- *What actually constitutes the critical trauma.* A traditional psychodynamic perspective stresses separation-individuation problems arising from maternal punishment of autonomy, whereas an abuse perspective includes (a) the role of early abuse and neglect as it interferes with the formation of secure attachment, typically in combination with (b) the disruptive and overwhelming impacts of early sexual invasion and injury—requiring the development of enduring survival responses and strategies that later in the child's life will be called borderline symptoms.
- *The gender and role of the most traumagenic parent.* Although the traditional dynamic perspective focuses on the dysfunctional mother, most sexual abusers are males, in many cases father figures. This is not to discount the fact that the concomitant neglect thought to prime a "borderline" response necessarily involves all potentially available caretakers, including (most frequently) mothers.
- *The age at the critical trauma.* A traditional psychodynamic analysis focuses on the first 1 to 2 years of life, whereas the average survivor reports that he or she was first sexually abused between age 6 and 9. It is true, however, that "borderline" difficulties may be more prominent when sexual abuse (and neglect) occurs significantly earlier in life.
- *The reason for the "borderline" behavior.* An abuse perspective stresses the functional or survival-based aspects of so-called borderline behaviors, especially in terms of adaptation, self-disturbance, tension reduction, and avoidance, whereas these same behaviors are consider to be signs of character pathology in traditional psychodynamic thought.

- *The prognosis associated with the problem.* Borderline personality disorder is often considered to be relatively unresponsive to treatment,
  whereas abuse-focused therapy with such individuals appears to be
  helpful in many instances.

An interesting attempt to reconcile these two perspectives in favor
of traditional analytic theory was offered by Henderson (1983).
Although admitting the possibility that borderline individuals might
have histories of childhood sexual abuse, he suggested that "an
equally plausible conclusion" (i.e., other than the causal role of sexual abuse) was that these women developed borderline characteristics in early childhood and then later *sought out* incest as a result of
their character pathology (p. 37).

In contrast to writers such as Henderson, Kernberg, or Masterson,
the perspective offered in this book (and by writers such as Kroll
[1993] and Linehan [1993]) is that a significant proportion of cases
(although clearly not all) of borderline personality disorder arise
from early and extended childhood sexual victimization, often with
concurrent or antecedent emotional abuse and neglect. The psychic
injuries that arise from a sexually victimizing environment are well
established and do not rest solely on dynamics associated with dysfunctional parent-child interactions in the first 1 or 2 years of life.
Instead of stressing contingent "libidinal supplies and gratification"
by the inevitably disordered mother (see Caplan & Hall-McCorquodale [1985] for a discussion of "mother-blaming" in traditional psychiatric theory), a survivor-oriented perspective suggests that the
cognitive, affective, and interpersonal effects of early, severe child
abuse and neglect are sufficient to account for many cases of what
is referred to as borderline behavior.

False Memory Syndrome

Perhaps the latest version of the hysterical or borderline survivor
exists in the inappropriate application of what has been called false
memory syndrome (FMS). This label, applied to those who report
recovered memories of previously "repressed" or dissociated sexual abuse, was created by a group of individuals (the FMS Foundation) who were accused of sexual abuse themselves by their now
adult children. This group makes a claim common to many of those

accused (correctly or otherwise) of a serious crime: They did not do it, and the accuser must be malicious, psychologically disturbed, or mislead to make such an accusation. From the FMS perspective, such false reports usually arise from psychologically vulnerable and suggestible women exposed to therapists who—by virtue of malice, avarice, or incompetence—directly or indirectly implant false memories of abuse. This argument has been used by defense expert witnesses, perpetrators, and the media to discount the testimony of most of those who report recovered memories of childhood abuse. Before the misuse of this issue can be addressed, however, a separate concern also must be considered: that of iatrogenically based memory distortion or confabulation.

It is likely that some proportion of the membership of the FMS group *have been* falsely accused. Any given individual reporting previously repressed or dissociated memories may be prey to the same afflictions found in the rest of the human race, including psychosis, confusion, desperation, greed, suggestibility, and intentional or unconscious misrepresentation. Further, some individuals who have been severely abused as children are, as adults, subject to dissociative symptoms, cognitive distortions, self-difficulties, and other abuse-related disturbances that can decrease, if not nullify, the accuracy of their reports.

In addition, it is likely that a small subset of mental health clients are "Grade 5 Syndrome" (Spiegel & Speigel, 1978) or "fantasy-prone" (Lynn & Rhue, 1988) individuals. Such people are reported to be highly imaginative, hypnotizable, suggestible, and prone to dissociation. Although more must be learned about this group, including the developmental antecedents of this personality pattern, it seems possible that such individuals would be especially prone to memory confabulation during exploratory psychotherapy.

Beyond client dynamics, and certainly more telling for the abuse field, there is little question that some clinicians have engaged in poor if not harmful "therapy," including attempting to convince clients that they have "repressed" abuse that has not, in fact, occurred. Through the inappropriate application of hypnosis or drug-assisted interviews, or as a result of overly directive verbal interventions, such clinicians may inadvertently lead susceptible clients (especially those suffering from "Grade 5" dynamics, dissociative disorders, and/or impaired self-functioning, as described later in this chapter) to believe things that have little or no basis in fact. This is not "recovered memory ther-apy," however, as some FMS advocates have suggested; involvement in authoritarian or overly directive approaches to treatment, whether involving "memory recovery" or not, is simply bad therapy (Briere, 1995a; Enns et al., 1995).

In this regard, it is important to acknowledge that people who have been falsely accused by those with grossly inaccurate or con-fabulated memories are victims as well. It would be inappropriate to discount their legitimate concerns and rights to redress by brand-ing them as inherently part of the backlash against survivors (Lind-say, 1995). To the extent that therapeutic errors produce or underlie false accusations against innocent individuals, the wronged parties deserve personal and legal redress, and certainly have the right to organize against those whose malpractice has harmed them.

Conversely, as noted by Enns et al. (1995) "it is also important to acknowledge that the overwhelming proportion of adult reports of adult survivors are based on significant and tangible human suffer-ing" (p. 203). The question, then, may not be whether recovered memory reports are all false or all true, but instead whether false memories can occur without negating the existence of truly recov-ered ones (Briere, 1995).

It is my clinical impression, supported by a growing body of re-search, that many (although not all) survivor reports of previously un-available abuse memories represent actual occurrences. To the extent that this is true, there exists a certain unpleasant irony: By negating true accounts of sexual abuse, our culture may be accomplishing exactly what it discounts in the survivor: "Repressing" or wishing away things that are too painful to tolerate in conscious awareness. Thus, although some unknown minority of repressed memory complaints are proba-bly invalid, the broad attacks on all of those reporting delayed (or of late, even always remembered) memories is unfair, at best.

Apropos of the earlier sections of this chapter, some critics have linked traditional Oedipal notions of hysterical female incest striv-ings with the newer "false memory" approach. For example, FMS proponent and child psychiatrist Richard Gardner posits:

> In our society, where the incest taboo is quite strong, little girls have to learn that their fathers are off limits when it comes to the expres-

sion and gratification of their sexual feelings. The suppression and repression of such feelings may produce some clinical and behavioral squelching, but they may press for release nonetheless. One way of dealing with them is via the mechanism of projection. In this way the individual is saying, "it is not I who harbor strong sexual desires toward my father, it is he who has strong sexual desires toward me." The next step is to have the fantasy that these desires were realized in reality. (1992, p. 178)

Rather than confronting this Oedipal delusion, Dr. Garner maintains, "sex abuse 'experts' are sprouting up in every field, coming out from under every stone, and suddenly appearing from behind every tree" (p. 653). In a similar vein, Gardner states "What better way to wreak vengeance on men than to become a therapist and use one's patients to act out one's morbid hostility" (p. 654).

Other FMS proponents (Loftus & Ketcham, 1994; Wakefield & Underwager, 1992) suggest that therapists essentially take advantage of gullible and easily mislead women clients by convincing them they have been abused. Although many clinicians would have little problem with a more circumscribed version of this analysis (i.e., in terms of specific instances of identifiable therapeutic malpractice), the FMS assumption is that almost *all* recovered memory reports implicitly represent this phenomenon—that there are thousands of corrupt or negligent therapists and, presumably, many more thousands of easily led women. In this way, both client and therapist are blamed for the invariably "false" accusation: the client for being hysterical and/or easily convinced of falsehoods, and the therapist for cynically or incompetently implanting false memories in the first place. Partially in response, the embattled abuse therapist cries "backlash" and angrily responds with equivalent vitriol.

Ultimately, the inappropriate use of the false memory defense serves to both invalidate true cases of recovered memory and, by virtue of its indiscriminate use, to reduce clinicians' nondefensive awareness of actual instances of memory confabulation and inappropriate therapeutic technique. At the same time, clinical errors that result in memory distortion create victims of both accuser and accused, and provide vivid examples of "false memory" and therapeutic incompetence for the FMS position.

CONCLUSION

Together, the labels of "hysteria," "borderline personality disorder," and "false memory syndrome" reflect the difficulties associated with understanding aberrant behavior in a culture that has long avoided the etiology of that behavior. Absent an understanding of the impacts of sexual abuse and the coping strategies that must be marshaled to survive such injury, the effects of child maltreatment are often interpreted as evidence of psychopathology. As a result, survivors who present as dramatically dysfunctional, self-destructive, alienated, or, for example, as having "suddenly remembered" things others assume they never would have forgotten do so in a contextual vacuum. Because the roots of their behavior are widely discounted by our culture, survivors' responses often appear to have no basis in reality: to be, by definition, irrational and pathological. As disordered and irrational beings, the explanations they offer for such behavior (e.g., "I was molested as a child") are easily discounted (even derided in some cases) and seen as further evidence of psychological disturbance. In this way, our culture often succeeds in marginalizing those who carry evidence of our own sins: our willingness to permit the wholesale sexual victimization of our children.

This analysis does not discount the considerable dysfunction of some survivors, or the likelihood that some reports of "repressed" memories are fallacious. Instead, it recognizes that the same culture that permits child abuse constructs our understanding of that abuse and its effects. In other words, a system dysfunctional enough to support the sexual victimization of over a fifth of its children might be expected to label its victims as secretly desiring abuse (the Oedipal approach), as manipulative and untrustworthy (the borderline analysis), or as unwitting liars (the false memory perspective). Given these social forces, the clinician must especially strive to view the survivor without socially constructed blinders, to see him or her in the context of his or her history. This more phenomenological perspective does not entirely discount traditional clinical and social understanding of the sexual abuse survivor, but, at the same time, it does not necessarily accept them as entirely objective truths.

The Core Effects
of Severe Abuse

3

As opposed to the enumeration of individual abuse effects found in chapter 1, and the potentially misleading social and psychiatric interpretation of abuse-related issues outlined in chapter 2, this chapter presents a broader theoretical analysis of the experience and impacts of sexual victimization. In addition, it links these phenomena to theories of "borderline" (and, to a lesser extent, "histrionic") symptom development. This more phenomenological perspective will be referred to as *core effects:* those impacts of sexual victimization thought to underlie the clinical problems or symptoms of abuse survivors, some of which relate to what is often referred to as personality disorder or character pathology. Although these expressions of trauma appear to be especially relevant to early-onset, chronic sexual abuse, the reader will undoubtably recognize aspects of these impacts in victims of severe physical and emotional abuse, and neglect as well.

Clinical experience, in combination with the abuse literature cited in chapter 1, suggests that the core impacts of severe or extended sexual victimization in childhood may be divided into several overlapping areas that underlie the survivor's clinical presentation. Each of these metaeffects is thought to be the direct result of traumatic interruptions of normal childhood development, such that the child's early personality is shaped by adaptation to victimization

51

and posttraumatic stress rather than solely in response to the usual environmental challenges and demands. These childhood responses are thought to elaborate and generalize over time, eventually resulting in chronic, seemingly maladaptive patterns of perception and behavior in adulthood. For the purposes of this discussion, these are referred to as (a) other-directedness, (b) chronic perception of danger, (c) negative self-perception, (d) "negative specialness," (e) conditional reality, (f) avoidance, (g) impaired self-functioning and tension reduction, and (h) posttraumatic intrusion.

CORE EFFECTS

Other-Directedness

The early life experiences of the severe sexual abuse survivor—especially in the case of intrafamilial victimization—are often characterized by invasion, exploitation, sudden and unpredictable dangers, and an overwhelming lack of security or safety. Faced with the frightening oxymoron of dangerous caretakers, the abused child may figuratively exist in what Louise Armstrong (1983) called "the family war zone." Such experiences can deprive the child of any real sense of control or self-determination, and often involves threats and acts of physical violence. Briere and Runtz (1987) found, for example, that of 133 psychotherapy clients who reported childhood histories of sexual abuse, 77% had experienced oral, anal, or vaginal penetration as a child, and 56% reported concomitant physical violence. In her book *The Secret Trauma: Incest in the Lives of Girls and Women*, sociologist Diana Russell (1986) quotes one woman's story:

> He got me out of bed and put me in his bed with him. He said if I hollered he would smother me with his pillow. He was kissing me and I started to fight him off, but he was a big strong man. He started feeling all over me, my breasts and my genitals. He took his fingers and forced them into my vagina. Then he started to force his penis into me. He got part of the way in when I remembered that my mother kept a hammer under the bed. I reached down, got it, and hit him on the head with it. (p. 239)

In such an atmosphere the victim of sexual or physical abuse quickly learns that safety is predicated on hypervigilance. She or he may become expert at reading the slightest nuance in the abuser because rapid and correct assessment of the perpetrator's psychological state may allow the victim either to (a) avoid or forestall an abuse incident by escaping in some manner, or (b) placate or fulfill the abuser's needs before a more aversive consequence ensues. Within the abuser's seemingly total control, the child may struggle to become "better" and "better," ultimately defining his or her own intrinsic value by the extent to which punishment or maltreatment can be avoided or the abuser can be pleased (note that because the abuse continues in most cases, the child can rarely achieve the goal of "goodness"). The survivor also learns that safety is predicated on constant vigilance to the (dangerous) external world.

The conclusions that one is only as good as powerful others see one to be, and only as safe as one's own vigilance allows, can produce a generalized sense of other-directedness wherein the survivor comes to rely on the reactions of people outside of herself as a basis for safety and self-esteem. This external locus may result in later "histrionic" or "borderline" hypersensitivity to others' negative opinions, a tendency to avoid threatening situations, and the belief that one must engage in a variety of pleasing or other-gratifying behaviors to be valued and, by extension, to survive. If one is rejected or found wanting, one is bad or unworthy, a perception that can result in intensely negative affects and feelings—especially in the context of interpersonal relationships.

The understanding of reality as externally determined also places survivors at significant risk from those who would exploit them or, ironically, treat them. Regarding the latter, the psychotherapist must recognize that what she or he presents as truth (e.g., through depth interpretations or advice) may have greater immediate salience for the former abuse victim than for some other clients because the survivor may have a less complete internal model of reality from which to evaluate therapist statements. As many of those who work with sexual abuse survivors will attest, this relative absence of self-reference is especially problematic when the sexually abused client is seen by an authoritarian clinician, who may convince the survivor that she fantasized the abuse, has false memories (or repressed ones), or that she sought out childhood victimization as a result of Oedipal sexual strivings.

Thus, the net effects of the radical other-directedness of many abuse survivors may include (a) hypersensitivity and extreme emotional reactivity to others (e.g., the affective instability and overreaction to minor interpersonal events described in the DSM-IV and elsewhere), especially in the face of rejection or abandonment, (b) suggestibility or malleability when confronted with the expectations or demands of peers or authority figures, in light of the survivor's poor sense of self-entitlement and ongoing training for subservience, (c) experience of isolation and neediness in the absence of internal support, and (d) boundary problems, arising from a relative inability to conceive of self without reference to others, and the reverse.

Chronic Perception of Danger

Given the salience of maltreatment and invasion in the survivor's early environment, the abuse victim's understanding of life must necessarily include such themes. Specifically, the child developing in an abusive context often makes important attributions or assumptions regarding the dangerousness of others, the likelihood of further injury or victimization, and the justness of the world. As noted earlier, these assumptions have been referred to as "cognitive distortions" because from the clinician's perspective, they are not grounded in accurate perceptions of current reality. Briefly stated, the survivor of severe abuse tends to perceive the world as dangerous and unjust, and his or her continued existence as tenuous. From this perspective, the child grows to view survival as the ultimate goal of life. This understanding of danger as a constant and survival as a daily task can produce a specific sense of desperation in the abuse victim: one that may be overlooked by the outside observer who sees no objective reason for distress.

Because they have found that the world is not necessarily or typically fair, and that betrayal is possible if not inevitable, some survivors learn to "look out for Number One" in any way possible—in behaviors ranging from prostitution to violence, or manipulativeness to serving as a "doormat" for powerful others. This understanding of human relationships as an adversarial process can produce a somewhat paradoxical dynamic: The survivor may become highly invested in control as a result of chronic feelings of helplessness. He or she may be, in some ways, strongly authoritarian: going "one down" when necessary, striving to be "one up" when possible, but almost always defining his actions in terms of control or power—a necessary perspective for one who must survive a hostile environment. Thus, for example, seductiveness becomes a way to influence dangerous, powerful others, and passivity serves to reassure such beings that their rule will not be challenged.

Contact with survivors who especially embody the qualities described in this section (e.g., "street kids," adolescent prostitutes, or "manipulative" patients) can suggest a sense of hardness or undue cynicism, qualities that may be perceived by others as evidence of toughness or incorrigibility. It is important that the clinician instead understands these behaviors as not freely chosen but rather as the logical extension of the survivor's view of himself or herself and the world.

Negative Self-Perception

Various parts of this book describe the low self-esteem or poor self-concept of the sexual abuse survivor. Such a relatively mild term does not embody the true extent of self-derogation experienced by some severely abused individuals, however. A more appropriate term might be self-hatred, for two reasons. First, it more accurately describes the extent of self-loathing seen in many survivors of severe sexual victimization. Some former sexual abuse victims, for example, report turning the mirrors in their homes to the wall so that, as one woman put it, "I won't have to be reminded of who or what I am," whereas others describe their bodies as disgusting or their minds as stupid. Other survivors describe elaborate self-mutilatory rituals designed to reduce the pervasive sense of guilt and badness they carry (what one client referred to as "my original sin").

The term *self-hatred* also implies introjection. To hate oneself is somewhat paradoxical: Hatred is most often thought of as an affect directed toward others. To hate oneself, therefore, implies a split of some sort: the one who is hateful and the one doing the hating. In the case of the sexual abuse survivor (as well as victims of other types of more extreme abuse), the "hating" part no doubt arises from the abuse process, where the victim incorporates from others the notion that she or he is essentially bad. Also implicit in hatred, however, is anger. Those we hate we often desire to harm. These combined qualities of self-dislike and the desire to harm one's self may arise from a variety of abuse-related processes, as described subsequently.

Finkelhor (1979a) has cited "stigmatization" as an abuse-specific basis for some survivor's negative self-perception. This term refers to the message the child directly receives from her or his abuser during or after victimization (e.g. "you are a whore," "you deserved every minute of it," or "you asked for it), or roughly equivalent communications when the abuse is discovered or addressed by others (e.g., the victim blaming often engaged in by parents, the police, or the courts). These direct sources of disconfirmation, involving verbal statements or labels, are often internalized by the child, ultimately becoming part of his or her self-image.

In contrast to such direct inputs, the victim also comes to devalue herself during the *process* of abuse. Based on the disclosures of many clinically depressed survivors, it appears that self-blame also arises from early attempts by the child to make sense of her or his victimization (Silver, Boon, & Stones, 1983). Specifically, the child who is faced with painful and intrusive events at the hands of an adult is, to some extent, forced to accept one of two possibilities: either (a) "this grown-up is hurting me because he or she is bad," or "I am being hurt because I am bad." This *abuse dichotomy* is likely to be resolved in favor of the child's own badness, given the many social (and abuser-delivered) messages that (a) adults know best and are inherently right when their views collide with a child's, (b) sometimes unpleasant things are done to you for your own good, and (c) adults sometimes rightfully hurt kids as punishment for things children have done wrong. In addition, from the child's perspective, the notion that one's own parents or caretakers are bad or dangerous may be frightening enough for any such thoughts to be denied or suppressed.

"Negative Specialness"

Despite the self-hatred of many sexual abuse survivors, there may be a paradoxical, almost magical sense of power—the ability to do bad. This sense arises, in part, from the early injunction to the child not to tell, that disclosure of the abuse may result in the breakup of the family, the arrest of the perpetrator, or some other catastrophic outcome. The perpetrator may also blame the abuse on the victim, telling her that some illicit quality about her (e.g., her sexuality, attractiveness, or seductiveness) rendered him incapable of restraining himself. The victim's experience of having a seemingly profound impact on an otherwise all-powerful being through sin and secrecy—in the general context of extreme powerlessness—can seem a central lesson to her about at least one route to efficacy or power.

In this way, the growing survivor may develop a belief in his or her own specialness regarding individuals in power. This specialness, however, is usually confined to sexual or sexualized interactions, and is often seen by the survivor as further confirmation of the badness in herself and in the object of her power. As expressed with considerable disgust by a former teenage prostitute who was trying to succeed in a "straight" job with an especially controlling supervisor: "When it's the worst, I always remind myself: This guy isn't any different from any other guy; you can always _____ him, they all want to screw you. They're all pigs who want what you've got."

> Angela is a 27-year-old office worker was brought to the attention of her Employee Assistance program by her manager. She willingly starts counseling with a social worker after requesting (and receiving) a male therapist. She reports in her second session that she was forced to "make love" with her father, beginning at age 8, and her two brothers at age 14. She still "goes out" (has sex) with her oldest brother (now age 32) on occasion, usually when he arrives at her apartment intoxicated. Angela frankly informs her therapist, "I'm not really good at much besides sex," and later asks if he "likes" her. She states in a challenging way that she has a "strange power over men" and that "I always get what I want." Her demeanor during therapy is what many clinicians would call seductive, although the therapist in this instance correctly discerned an underlying anger and brittle desperation rather than actual sexual interest. Angela appears paradoxically reassured when the social worker states that sex has no place in the client–therapist relationship, although she comments, "Since when?" (On questioning, she refuses to identify specifically any therapist who may have had sexual contact with her). She is

eventually transferred to a woman therapist experienced in the treatment of sexual abuse victims, to whom she confides that "sex isn't an
experience, it's a tool."

This sense of power to control others through sex may cause some
survivor behavior to be seen as narcissistic by psychotherapists,
especially when the former victim is able to mask her or his self-
hatred and insecurity. The facade of cynicism and streetwise arro-
gance may be especially important to the survivor, who needs to feel
control over at least some portion of his or her interactions with others, if only those related to further sexual exploitation. More deeply,
this "power to do bad" is partially an exercise in self-hatred that
may increase over time as a self-fulfilling prophesy: I do bad because I am bad, and I am bad because of what I do.

Conditional Reality

The victim of severe sexual abuse (as well as the survivor of
extensive physical or emotional abuse) often has been deprived of
the experience of internally held truth. Through the necessity of
viewing others as critically important to avoid greater pain or danger as well as the effects of early dissociation and attachment disruption described in a later section, the survivor may fail to develop
a personal map of reality that is stable across different interpersonal
situations. This paucity of reliable internal landmarks means that
the survivor may view reality as a relative abstraction that is ultimately conditional as opposed to concrete. From this perspective,
what one perceives to be true may not be true (e.g., the perpetrator's
statements that "I'm doing this because I love you," "You made me
do this," or "That never happened"); it can be verified or defined
only by others.

The flip side of this process can manifest as "pathological lying"
for a minority of survivors, given their understanding that reality
is not, in fact, real, but rather a construct that can be molded or
altered according to external contingencies. Lies become, under this
condition, both a survival technique (as the child learns that mis-
representing facts or "the truth" can sometimes forestall abusive or
punitive behaviors from others) and a problem (as the survivor

becomes increasingly unclear about where the lies end and reality begins). In most cases, the personal contingencies for such misrepresentations include the need to escape pain, to be liked or respected by a given individual, or to be someone better than who one "really" is.

> Fernando is an 13-year-old boy who was referred to a school psychologist for chronic lying. Reports from his teachers as well as his behavior during a diagnostic interview indicate that this young man makes up elaborate stories on a regular basis without obvious provocation. These stories are often internally contradictory or clearly false, yet it often appears that Fernando believes his fabrications as he relates them (although he rarely remembers them later). Most of these "lies" are self-aggrandizing or self-justifying, although occasionally they are about unrelated events or people. Overall, there is a sad, ingratiating quality about this boy that causes people to pity him at the same time that they castigate him for his lack of truthfulness. School records indicate that Fernando lives in a group home, where he was placed after his father was arrested for involving him in child prostitution and pornography. It appears, however, that the crimes for which his father was incarcerated were only the "tip of the iceberg" relative to the years of extreme emotional neglect and both physical and sexual abuse that Fernando experienced from his father.

Although the weakness of a stable reality representation for some survivors of severe sexual abuse may underlie a variety of symptoms and behaviors, including "pathological" lying, poor boundaries, split-off ego states, and "Grade 5 Syndrome," most basically the problem is a disturbance of self. This is perhaps best described by a male adolescent who exclaimed in frustration during a juvenile hall interview, "Don't you understand? There's nobody inside here to hear what you say. I'm just empty. I just do what happens."

Heightened Ability to Avoid Distress

Withdrawal from stressful or aversion stimuli is a normal, adaptive human behavior. Clearly, it is neither helpful nor healthy for anyone to dwell on or confront every painful aspect of life—to do so would undoubtedly interfere with successful daily functioning. As a result, most people have developed ways to circumvent or ignore things they otherwise might find distressing. This core effect refers to the overdevelopment of these coping strategies in the survivor of severe abuse, who has had to become an expert in avoidance to survive his or her history psychologically. Unfortunately, such proficiency ultimately can become maladaptive: Although avoidance can decrease anxiety temporarily, it rarely solves problems and (as noted in chapter 5) it often interferes with the normal processing and resolution of traumatic stress.

Avoidance refers to conscious, intentional behavior designed to reduce contact with stressful phenomena, and less consciously chosen defenses used to reduce anxiety and other negative affects. Originally used by the survivor to minimize interactions with abusive individuals (e.g., staying away from home, feigning sickness, or avoiding certain activities in the presence of the perpetrator), conscious avoidance behaviors may later interfere with normal functioning or access to helpers. For example, the survivor who has learned to procrastinate, make excuses, or "disappear" when confronted with an abusive situation may use these same strategies to miss psychotherapy sessions, fail to acknowledge significant life problems, avoid Alcoholics Anonymous meetings, or keep from attending classes or work.

As opposed to classic behavioral avoidance, denial involves a somewhat less conscious attempt to underestimate, not think about, or cognitively avoid awareness of threatening events. Survivors of severe abuse are prone to using such coping behaviors as a result of their reinforcement in the past—for example, the relief felt by the child victim when she was able to block complete awareness of the reality and horror of her sexual abuse. Survivor denial can lead to increased gullibility and susceptibility to injurious activities or revictimization because the individual may specifically overlook warning signals (e.g., potentially threatening stimuli) that might lead others to avoid specific persons or situations. Denial may additionally allow survivors to underestimate the extent of their victimization and its long-term effects, thereby supporting avoidance of psychotherapy or other help-focused (but anxiety-provoking) interventions.

Thus, although abuse-related denial may temporarily reduce dysphoria, one of the down sides of this defense for the survivor is that attenuating anxiety can disarm early warning systems that might otherwise alert her or him to danger. Herein lies what seems to be a contradiction: How can the survivor be hypervigilant to danger and yet be unaware of it because of overdeveloped avoidance mechanisms? This inconsistency is more apparent than real, however, because (a) most survivors predominate in one mode or the other—some tend toward fearful apprehension, whereas others are prone to denial (see Byrne, 1961, for a well-known personality theory that divides most people into "sensitizers" and "repressors"), and (b) even in those survivors for whom denial is a major defense, there is often an underlying tension, hypervigilance, and emotional brittleness, which appears to reflect only partially inhibited fearful awareness. This impression of fragility may be accompanied by a facade of extreme positivity (e.g., "I feel wonderful," "Everything's great," or "I had a perfect childhood"), as is often described for "histrionic" clients.

The most extreme (and least conscious) form of avoidance is that of dissociative amnesia. As the term is typically used, amnesia refers to an unconscious dissociation or splitting off of memories from awareness to avoid the painful affects that would otherwise accompany such recollections. DSM-IV notes that

> Dissociative amnesia most commonly presents as a retrospectively reported gap or series of gaps in recall for aspects of the individual's life history. These gaps are usually related to traumatic or extremely stressful events. (American Psychiatric Association, 1994, p. 478)

This amnestic response is not specific to sexual abuse survivors; probably all humans are capable of "forgetting" things that we are unable to confront fully. In this regard, recent reviews of the literature catalog a wide variety of case reports and studies published over the years that document psychogenic amnesia in war veterans, victims of violence, and others exposed to extreme stress (Lowenstein, 1993). What merits the inclusion of this dissociative defense here is its extreme development in some severely abused individuals. Specifically, some survivors appear to have the ability to avoid remembering the most painful aspects of early childhood victimization. Such behavior may be understood as learned, cognitive solutions to the overwhelmingly painful affect associated with memories of severe childhood trauma.

As noted earlier, the notion of amnesia for child abuse has been the subject of considerable controversy. Ofshe and Waters (1994), for example, virtually deny dissociative amnesia ever occurs, despite the description of this response in the last three Diagnostic and Statistical Manuals of the American Psychiatric Association (DSM-III, DSM-III-R, and DSM-IV). In a similar vein, the title of Loftus and Ketcham's (1994) latest book is *The Myth of Repressed Memories,* thereby contending that reports of amnesia are inevitably without any basis in reality. Interestingly, however, several FMS advocates and recovered memory critics do appear to acknowledge the possibility that at least some postabuse amnesia may occur (Gardner, 1992; Lindsay, 1995; Rogers, 1992; Wakefield & Underwager, 1992).

Although the current research is methodologically insufficient to establish the incidence of abuse-related amnesia definitively (Briere, 1992b), and some reports of recovered sexual abuse memories are likely to be distorted or even entirely fictitious, the gradually accumulating clinical and research database suggests that impaired memory for trauma is a significant problem for abuse survivors (Enns et al., 1995), one that is not easily discounted.

In this regard, several studies suggest that some proportion of adults sexually abused as children have less than complete knowledge of their abuse experiences. Herman and Schatzow (1987) reported that 64% of 53 women undergoing group therapy for sexual abuse trauma indicated some level of amnesia for their abuse. Reports of memory impairment were associated with more violent abuse that began earlier in life. Briere and Conte (1993) more recently found that of 450 women and men who were in outpatient treatment for sexual-abuse–related difficulties, 59% reported having had some period before age 18 when they had no knowledge of being abused. Both Herman and Schatzow (1987) and Briere and Conte (1993) found that self-reported abuse-related amnesia was associated with severer and extensive abuse that occurred at a relatively earlier age.

Although critics themselves of the concept of recovered memories, Loftus and colleagues recently published a study of 105 women who were in treatment for substance abuse, and found that 19% reported some point when they had no memories of what they later recalled as sexual abuse (Loftus, Polonsky, & Fullilove, 1994). Loftus et al suggest, however, that this phenomenon may have been due to "normal forgetting" or merely of not having thought about the abuse for some period. Offering a perhaps culturally insensitive example of the latter, Loftus et al suggested that a woman in this sample of inner-city, predominantly Black low-income, single mothers might have thought "I spent one nice summer in Europe where I didn't think about the abuse at all" (p. 81) and thus may have inappropriately endorsed having forgotten then remembering a child abuse history.

Three additional studies have examined the possibility of recovered memories but have used nonclinical samples. This focus on nonpsychotherapy subjects reflects the appropriate concerns voiced by critics that studies using clinical subjects may not be good tests of the recovered memory hypothesis—because of either the influence of mental health problems on accurate reporting or the potential bias associated with being treated by therapists who may already believe in recovered memories.

Feldman-Summers and Pope (1994) studied a national sample of 330 psychologists and found that—of those reporting childhood sexual abuse—40.5% described some period when they had less or no memory of the abuse. Approximately one half of these psychologists reported that their memory recovery did not occur in the context of psychotherapy. Elliott and Briere (1995) examined self-reported delayed recall of sexual abuse in a random sample of 505 individuals from the general population. Forty-two percent of those reporting a childhood history of sexual abuse also described some period when they had less memory of the abuse than they did at the point of data collection. Being in therapy, sex, race, income, and other demographic variables were not significant predictors of reporting recovered sexual abuse memories.

Finally, in a methodological improvement over the preceding studies, Williams (1994) followed up a nonclinical sample of women who, as children, had been seen in an urban emergency room (ER) with a primary complaint of having been sexually abused. She interviewed these subjects approximately 18 to 20 years later—without indicating that she knew about their childhood ER visit—and asked them whether they had ever been sexually abused as children. Approximately 38% of this sample reported not having been sexually abused in any way similar to what the ER records described. Although it cannot be proved that these women did not just deny abuse of which they were well aware, such data—especially in combination with the retrospective studies—suggest that defensive avoidance mechanisms may produce complete or partial amnesia for abuse in some individuals.

Although these research findings appear to document instances of total amnesia for abuse, clinical experience suggests that dissociative amnesia is often not complete, nor is it necessarily permanent. Instead, access to trauma-relevant information may wax and wane over time as a function of stress and level of internal resources, and often can be triggered by environmental events that are especially reminiscent of the original trauma. Such recall may take the form of sudden sensory flashbacks to a painful experience, or as more complex and integrated chunks of material that most would define as "memories" per se (Elliott & Briere, 1995). In its most typical presentation, this avoidance activity results in patchy or incomplete memories of the abuse, so that the survivor may not recall exactly what happened, while nevertheless having a negative emotional reaction to it. This absence of hard facts may be used by the survivor—as well as others in her life—to discount the importance or truthfulness of her abuse. Such dissociation may also interfere with therapy because the former abuse victim may be less able to accept something that he or she cannot clearly or completely recall.

Therapy that addresses available traumatic memory also may aid in the recovery of thus far unavailable memories. Specifically, cognitive processing and affective desensitization of available traumatic material (as outlined in chapter 5) may reduce the overall level of stress the survivor is experiencing, thereby lessening the need for avoidance defenses as primitive as simply "not knowing." Thus, it is possible for someone to enter therapy with partial or unavailable memories of childhood trauma and yet to leave treatment at some later point with specific memories of abuse—an event that might appear to an outside observer as evidence of therapy having created abuse memories. However, as noted in chapter 5, the fact that previously unavailable memories sometimes emerge as a side effect of effective abuse-focused therapy does not mean that (a) memory recovery "should" occur or is absolutely required for successful therapy outcome, or (b) that badly done therapy cannot confuse the issue by capitalizing on client suggestibility and producing invalid or contaminated memories.

Impaired Self-Functioning and Tension-Reduction Behavior

Thus far, much of the material in this book has been devoted to posttraumatic, cognitive, and behavioral, or defense-related effects of abuse. There is another general area, however, in which childhood sexual abuse can have substantial effects: on that of the Self. The Self may be considered a collection of internal skills and capacities that, among other things, determine the extent to which trauma-related distress is accommodated to or becomes overwhelming. Although a variety of self-capacities and resources have been posited (McCann & Pearlman, 1990), three are especially important to the individual's response to aversive events: identity, boundary, and affect regulation.

Identity refers to a consistent sense of personal existence, of an internal locus of conscious awareness. A strong sense of personal identity is helpful in the face of potentially traumatic events because it allows the individual to respond from a secure internal base, wherein challenging stimuli can be readily organized and contextualized without excessive confusion or disorientation. Individuals whose sense of identity is less stable or who "lose track" of themselves in the face of upsetting events may easily become overwhelmed; they may become less internally organized and may fragment at those very times when awareness of their own needs, perspectives, entitlement, and goals are most necessary.

Boundary is closely related to identity, in that it refers to an individual's awareness of the demarcation between self and other. People said to have poor or weak boundaries have difficulty knowing where their identities, needs, and perspectives end and others' begin, such that they either allow others to intrude on them, or they inappropriately transgress on others (Elliott, 1994). An absence of boundaries when confronted with a stressor can reduce the individual's ability to negotiate interpersonal interactions, leading to, for example, difficulties in self-other discrimination, effective help seeking, and self-assertion in the face of victimization. The boundary-impaired victim of a traumatic assault may also be less aware of his or her rights to safety, leading to inappropriate acceptance of being victimized.

The third self-function, that of *affect* regulation, has been viewed as important to the individual's management of traumatic experiences and negative internal states (Briere, 1996; Linehan, 1993). Affect regulation may be divided into two subfunctions: affect modulation and affect tolerance. The first refers to the individual's ability to engage in internal activities that in some way allow him or her to reduce or change painful emotionality (McCann & Pearlman, 1990). Activities thought to assist in affect modulation include self-soothing, positive self-talk, placing upsetting events in perspective, and self-distraction. Affect tolerance, conversely, refers to the individual's relative ability to experience sustained negative affects without having to resort to external activities that distract or soothe, or avoidance through the use of dissociation or psychoactive substances. For example, people with good affect tolerance may be able to experience considerable frustration, anxiety, or anger without engaging in tension-reduction behaviors, such as aggression, self-mutilatory activities, sexual "acting out," or self-destructiveness.

Normal Development of Self-Functions

The self-functions described previously are thought to arise from normal childhood development, primarily in the first years of life (Cole & Putnam, 1992). Identity and boundary awareness, for example, are likely to unfold in the context of normal parent-child attachment experiences. As the child interacts in the context of one or more consistent, loving, and supportive caretakers, a sense of self in contradistinction to "other" develops. This sense of self incorporates the sustained and reliable positive responses of the caregiver, typically leading to self-esteem, self-efficacy, and a view of others and the interpersonal environment as essentially benign. In combination, these and related processes result in a sense of internal stability: a secure psychological base from which to interact with the world (Bowlby, 1988).

As the child develops in a generally positive (or at least good enough) environment, he or she nevertheless encounters a variety of surmountable obstacles or challenges—ranging from diaper rash to small frustrations to momentarily unavailable caretakers. In the context of sustained external security, the child learns to deal with the associated uncomfortable (but not overwhelming) internal states through trial and error, slowly building a progressively more sophisticated set of internal coping strategies as he or she grows and confronts increasingly more challenging and stressful experiences (Briere, 1996). At the same time, because the associated discomfort does not exceed the child's growing internal resources, he or she is able to become increasingly at home with some level of distress and is able to tolerate greater levels of emotional pain. This growing affective competence is likely to be self-sustaining: As the individual becomes better able to modulate and tolerate distress or dysphoria, such discomfort becomes less destabilizing, and the individual is able to seek more challenging and complex interactions with the environment without being derailed by concomitant increases in stress and anxiety.

Effects of Abuse on Self-Functions

Because the development of self-capacities and -functions occurs during childhood, child maltreatment is an unfortunately potent source of later self-difficulties (Cole & Putnam, 1992; Elliott, 1994d). Although self-functioning is also affected by early neglect, early childhood sexual abuse may produce long-standing difficulties in the self-domain (Friedrich, 1994, 1996). In this regard, sexual victimization during early childhood can be injurious by virtue of its ability to disrupt normal development and preclude the development of the self-functions outlined previously.

Implicit in the normal attachment process is the child's growing sense of safety and security—a base from which he or she can remain maximally "open" to experience, and from which he or she can explore intrapersonal and interpersonal environments and develop increasingly sophisticated self-skills (Bowlby, 1988). In the case of child abuse, however, safety is diminished or disappears alto-gether. Faced with parental intrusion or violence, the child may develop an avoidant style of relating, wherein he or she psycholog-ically limits or avoids attachment interactions with a given abusive caretaker. Although this defense protects the child, to some extent, from pain, it also tends to reduce his or her responsivity to any pos-itive attachment stimuli that might be available in the environment. This response, in turn, further deprives the child of normal attach-ment-related learning, including the development of identity, boundary, and affect regulation skills and capacities.

It is likely that one of the primary ways in which the child avoids abuse-related distress is through dissociation, as noted earlier. Beyond its impacts on attachment, dissociation during early abuse is thought to reduce opportunities for learning how to tolerate painful affect without avoidance. Dissociation is also likely to pre-clude the need to develop other, more complex and conscious affect regulation skills. In the words of one survivor in treatment, "I spaced out [during] most of my childhood. I was never around to learn regular ways of dealing with hassles." This forced reliance on dissociation during early childhood thus motivates the continued need for dissociation and other primitive avoidance strategies later in life.

Finally, the other-directedness described earlier in this chapter may negatively impact the development of self-capacities. The growing child's proficiency at meeting the needs or avoiding the violence of the abuser exacts a price; The sustained and concentrated attention she or he must pay to a threatening external world inevitably pulls energy and attention away from the (internal) devel-opmental tasks of self-awareness and the acquisition of affect mod-ulation skills.

Development of Tension-Reduction Behavior

In the absence of sufficient self-capacities, the survivor must rely on dissociation or external ways of dealing with painful internal experience, especially when it is restimulated by current events. These external activities (e.g., compulsive sexual behavior, binging, or self-mutilation) are often seen as "acting out," "impulsivity," or—of late—as arising from "addictions." For the abuse survivor, however, such behaviors may best be understood as problem-solving behaviors in the face of extreme dysphoria and reduced self-functioning.

Tension-reduction behaviors are thought to work by providing temporary distraction, interrupting intrusive experiences, anesthetizing psychic pain, restoring a sense of control, temporarily "filling" perceived emptiness, communicating isolation and pain, or relieving guilt (Briere, 1992a). Because of the frequent effectiveness of such behaviors, a sense of calm and relief ensues for some period. Ultimately, the use of tension-reducing mechanisms in the future is reinforced through a process of negative reinforcement or avoidance learning; behavior that reduces pain is likely to be repeated in the presence of future pain.

Unfortunately for the survivor, although often immediately effective, such behavior is rarely adaptive in the long-term, leading to repeated cycles of tension reduction, subsequent calm, and the slow building of further tension and, ultimately, further tension reduction. In addition, to the extent that avoidance responses like tension reduction succeed, the survivor continues to be deprived of the opportunity to develop more sophisticated affect regulation techniques.

Posttraumatic Intrusion

Beyond its impacts on self-development, the violence of child abuse can produce posttraumatic intrusive symptoms, as described in chapter 1. Modern trauma theory suggests that the flashbacks, nightmares, rumination, and other intrusive symptoms of posttraumatic stress are triggered when traumatic experience stresses the individual by challenging the self's capacities to "handle" or integrate such stimuli (McCann & Pearlman, 1990). This may occur as a result of preexisting inadequate self-capacities or in the face of extreme trauma regardless of self resources.

Given that overwhelming stressors commonly produce repetitive intrusive experiences, an important question is what psychological purpose, if any, such painful and disruptive phenomena might serve. Integrating Horowitz's (1976, 1986) cognitive accommodation theory with behavioral exposure models and recent theories of emotional processing, I suggest that posttraumatic intrusion is an inborn self-healing activity (Briere, 1996). Specifically, symptoms, such as flashbacks, intrusive thoughts, traumatic preoccupation, and nightmares, may represent the mind's attempt to desensitize and integrate affectively laden material by repeatedly exposing itself to small, moderately distressing fragments of an otherwise overwhelming trauma (e.g., brief sensations, repetitive thoughts, or incomplete autobiographic memories) until the survivor "gets over it" and the material can recede from awareness. Because this occurs after the trauma, the intrusive material is not accompanied by actual danger (as was originally the case), and thus the posttraumatic distress associated with the traumatic memory eventually fades from lack of reinforcement. Further, the relief associated with emotional discharge (e.g., crying or raging) is likely to countercondition the distress normally associated with the material. From this perspective, flashbacks and related intrusive experiences; avoidant symptoms, such as numbing and cognitive disengagement; and intense expressions of emotional distress represent the mind's desensitization and processing activities more than they reflect underlying pathology.

Unfortunately, some survivors of severe child maltreatment (and later adult traumas) are not able to desensitize and accommodate trauma fully through intrusive reexperiencing of affects, memories, or cognitions alone, and hence present with chronic posttraumatic stress. This may occur because the severity of the trauma or the extent of impaired self-capacities motivates excessive use of cognitive and emotional avoidance strategies. This avoidance (e.g., dissociation), in turn, lessens the survivor's self-exposure to traumatic material, as well as decreasing the availability of the associated anxious arousal to habituation. In other words, posttraumatic dissociation and other defensive avoidance responses may reduce the effectiveness of the intrusion-desensitization process, leading to incomplete resolution of traumatic stress. In support of this notion, it appears that individuals who tend to avoid cognitive access to traumatic material suffer more psychological distress than do those with less avoidant tendencies (Wirtz & Harrell, 1987). This seeming competition between two relatively automatic trauma-related processes, intrusion and avoidance, will be considered in the upcoming chapters on treatment.

Summary

These first three chapters have described, in some detail, the potential long-term effects of childhood sexual victimization. It is important to recognize, however, that not all sexual abuse automatically confers major long-term psychological problems. There are many survivors in the general population who appear to have experienced relatively little distress as a result of their victimization and who report few long-term consequences. Additionally, because most adults molested as children did not receive appropriate therapy at the time, the sexual abuse literature is primarily concerned with the effects of *untreated* victimization. Thus, individuals who have received therapy for abuse as children may be less likely to present with post–sexual-abuse trauma in adulthood.

Nevertheless, there are many women and men whose childhood experiences were so destructive that they continue to suffer as adults. These experiences are described as severe in light of their power to overwhelm the victim's immediate self-resources and equilibrium. Thus, abuse severity is a somewhat relative notion in the sense that different victims may have greater or lesser abilities to resist injury—what may be overwhelming abuse for one person may be less destructive for another. Certain aspects of sexual abuse are especially likely to increase its impact, however, such as early onset, especially violent or intrusive acts, incest, or extended periods of victimization. Other concomitant or antecedent forms of child maltreatment (e.g., emotional neglect or physical abuse) also may exacerbate the effects of sexual abuse. People who have experienced these more extreme and complex events are often among those who come to psychotherapists for help—help that is not always forthcoming. The remainder of this book is concerned with describing a treatment philosophy and a variety of therapeutic techniques and approaches that may be helpful for such people.

Philosophy of Treatment 4

Having considered the major long-term effects and social context of childhood sexual victimization, the remainder of this book is devoted to treatment of the abuse survivor. A presentation of abuse effects and treatment techniques alone, however, does not necessarily result in therapeutic effectiveness—even for accomplished psychotherapists. Perhaps even more important than these technical aspects is the therapist's general orientation toward working with survivors of sexual victimization. For this reason, this chapter outlines a general philosophy of treatment—one that may be relevant to any work with abused or victimized individuals, but that is, nevertheless, specifically presented here in terms of the treatment of sexual abuse effects.

PHILOSOPHICAL PRINCIPLES

The Abuse Perspective

The primary axiom in work with former sexual abuse victims is intuitively obvious at this point: As opposed to other approaches, survivor-oriented therapy specifically considers the original abuse context to be one of the key issues in the treatment of abuse survivors, relating this early trauma to later and current experiences and behavior. Other aspects of the survivor's childhood are likely to have been destructive as well (e.g., attachment disruption, dysfunctional family dynamics, inconsistent or uncaring parenting, and psychological or physical abuse), often intensifying those symptoms specifically associated with the sexual abuse. As a result, the clinician must be attuned to the full breadth of the survivor's childhood experience rather than limiting his or her analysis solely to the technically sexual components of the client's sexual abuse experience.

Although the notion of attending to childhood issues may seem obvious to some when the client describes sexual abuse as the presenting problem, therapists may be less likely to consider abuse issues when (as is often the case) the survivor complains of more "garden variety" problems, such as depression, substance abuse, chronic self-destructiveness, or sexual dysfunction. In such cases, abuse disclosures are likely to be treated as less relevant to the problems at hand or as remote factors too distant to address. A survivor-oriented perspective, conversely, suggests that childhood molestation may be related to a variety of adolescent and adult mental health problems, and that therapeutic attention to such seemingly ancient events may nevertheless have a significant impact on current psychological functioning.

The issue often becomes: "What is abuse-related, and what is not?" Not all psychological problems are associated with sexual abuse, nor are all problems of abuse survivors a result of their childhood victimization. The therapist is counseled, in this regard, to (a) accurately assess the client's current difficulties, using appropriate psychological tests and sensitive interviewing techniques (Briere, in press, b); (b) inquire as to whether there was sexual abuse in childhood (and, if so, its extent, severity, and duration); and then (c) drawing on the relevant literature and clinical experience, evaluate which, if any, of the client's presenting problems may be related to his or her molestation history. In the event that a significant abuse-symptom relationship seems likely, the clinician should consider approaching those abuse-related problems from an abuse perspective, as outlined in subsequent chapters. Failure to do so (e.g., ignoring chronic incest in a "borderline" client) may doom the therapist's best efforts to relative failure because the etiological roots of the problem will not have been adequately addressed.

Conversely, if the survivor's presenting problems do not appear to be abuse related, or if they do but the client does not want to address sexual abuse, the therapist should not somehow force an abuse perspective on the client. Abuse-focused therapy requires the full permission and participation of the survivor to succeed, and can easily convey either insensitivity or authoritarian indifference when used inappropriately.

Question of Truth

Although in many cases, the well-meaning therapist may be willing to accept the relevance of abuse experiences to certain later psychological problems, there are often instances when the client's disclosure of molestation is disbelieved. This tendency to deny that sexual abuse took place may occur when the client presents with "histrionic" or "borderline" characteristics or behavior (e.g., those that are dramatic, sexualizing, or manipulative). In such instances, the therapist may assume that the abuse disclosure serves a secondary gain, intended primarily to accomplish increased credibility or greater attention, or that it reflects fantasy material or "primary process thinking" in a highly disturbed individual. As chapters 2 and 3 described, however, this sort of clinical presentation has been empirically and clinically associated with a history of childhood victimization. Given this conundrum, the clinician may be left with the question: "How do I know what happened, and what didn't?"

Some therapists have dealt with this ambiguity by constructing an internal list of what they believe to be truisms regarding abuse and then comparing the client's presentation to this list. Among these "truths" are the notions that (a) abuse disclosures should be accompanied by intense negative affect—the client should cry or show some other evidence of obvious psychological pain (yet should not be so emotional or upset as to appear histrionic); (b) the story should be consistent—there should be no major gaps in the recounting, and the major points should be consistent from disclosure to disclosure (but not so consistent as to appear rote); and

(c) the client should appear authentic—there should be no hidden agendas.

Unfortunately, these litmus tests for abuse are likely to be invalid. Molestation disclosures often precipitate—or occur in the context of—dissociation and other psychological defenses that allow the survivor to detach from, titrate, or somehow alter the painful affect associated with replaying an abuse memory. Such coping techniques may result in either little visible emotional response (e.g., affective blunting or seemingly mechanical renditions) or "inappropriate" responses, such as laughter, inordinate casualness, or intellectualization. Second, the survivor's unconscious attempts to deal with the painful affect surrounding victimization experiences may have generated periods of amnesia or confusion regarding the specifics of the abuse and may be associated with conflicting memories and perceptions. The client's continuing attempt to avoid the abuse (and thus render it nonexistent or at least unimportant) unfortunately may be all too successful in the short term, occasionally producing questions in the therapist's mind regarding the truth of the disclosure or the possibility of "false memories." Finally, sexual abuse often results in disturbed interpersonal functioning, such that the client's behavior in therapy (an intensely interpersonal and, therefore, threatening event) is likely to include some "gamesy," adversarial, or dysfunctional components.

More basically, the therapist must question himself or herself as to why the exact, "real" facts are so important in treating adults who report childhood molestation. In other areas of psychotherapy, it is often benignly assumed that clients' reports of past events—although frequently distorted by defenses and previous experiences—have some intrinsic validity, and the client is rarely cross-examined as to the detailed aspects of his or her historical account. Nevertheless, some therapists appear to be significantly invested in determining absolute truth or falsehood when the client issue is sexual victimization. It is in this regard that the clinician must examine his or her assumptions: Do I especially question the honesty of this disclosure in part because I have been trained (socially and professionally) to doubt reports of sexual victimization? Would I be significantly more comfortable if this were a false disclosure? To the extent that the answers are affirmative, resolution of the veracity question may ultimately become as much a therapist issue as a client one.

Some therapists appear invested in detecting the absolute truth of an abuse disclosure because they fear being tricked or "taken in," believing that such potential gullibility would reflect badly on them as clinicians. It is likely, however, that we are often misled, to some extent, by our clients—a nonmalicious state of affairs that generally does not sustain itself over the course of therapy or prove overwhelmingly destructive. Perhaps more important, it is probably rare that a given client seeks to create an entirely fictitious history during psychotherapy. It is possible, however, especially early in treatment, for a client with severe trauma to present with less than clear memories of what exactly transpired, or for memories to be contradictory or technically impossible (e.g., abuse that could not have occurred at that specific moment in time). Some survivors with frightening but incomplete memories may be driven to form premature closure—essentially "deciding" on an unconscious level to accept a specific version of a given hurtful occurrence rather than feeling the pain associated with injury compounded by uncertainty.

In my experience, frequently all that is required of the therapist at such times is to endorse the reality of the client's pain, as well as the general plausibility of his or her explanation for such distress (if, in fact, it is plausible), while giving her sustained permission and support to avoid a premature, definitive conclusion regarding what *exactly* happened. The general message is that the client is experiencing real pain, born of real occurrences, but that such pain and such frightful events often lead to defenses that block or distort access to "all the facts."

One of the times when the therapist must be especially concerned with the specific veracity of a given abuse report, however, is when the report has major impacts on other people, such as in lawsuits, criminal complaints, and so forth. For this reason, it is important to advise the confused or unclear client against actions outside of therapy until therapy has done what it can to clarify the relevant material. Thus, it is never appropriate for the therapist to attempt to force clarity on dissociated or distorted client memories in the interest of external justice. If the client (and, it is hoped, the therapist) has come to a natural point of understanding regarding who did what when, the client may appropriately choose to file a criminal or civil complaint. Any such decision to seek legal redress must be the client's, however, as opposed to being suggested or directed by the therapist.

Even when the client insists on a suit, however, I recommend that (a) the clinician counsel the client to consider carefully the fact that civil litigation is frequently unsuccessful in such instances, and often opens up the client's life (and his or her therapy records) to potentially traumatic scrutiny via the accused's right to discovery; and (b) the therapist not participate in the resultant court case, at least not as an expert witness on sexual abuse or as holder of absolute truth regarding the client (Briere, in press, a).

To summarize this difficult issue, the notion of truthfulness must hinge on the client's experience, while considering the subjectivity of that criterion. The stance of the therapist is to accept the generally truthful client's historical rendition as likely to be an approximate version of what he or she recollects, and to understand the role of therapy as a vehicle whereby greater clarity regarding the client's childhood may be accomplished as an epiphenomenon of psychological recovery.

Question of Responsibility

Just as the issue of truthfulness may come up for therapists working with sexual abuse survivors, another frequent question is in the area of responsibility. As described earlier, it is a common practice in our society to blame the victim, including in those instances when the victim is a child. Therapists are no more immune to this bias than other groups, although they may be in a position to do more harm as a result of it. This tendency to assign responsibility for abuse to the victim frequently manifests in psychotherapy as questions, such as: "What was your part in all this?;" "Didn't you get something out of it, though, for it to have gone on for so long"; or even "Deep down, didn't some part of you want it to happen/like it?"

These questions or statements often reflect the traditional Oedipal notion that children wish for sexual contact from adults and thus to some extent are responsible for any sexual interactions that subsequently transpire. We need only recall psychiatrist Henderson's statement that "the daughters *collude* in the incestuous *liaison* and play an active and even *initiating* role in establishing the pattern" (1975, p. 1356; emphasis added) to understand the extent to which the sexual abuse survivor may be blamed in mainstream mental health philosophy. Words, such as "collude," suggest a conspiracy between two equals, "initiating" goes further to place primary responsibility on the victim, and "liaison" implies that the abuse experience was an enjoyable, romantic affair rather than an act of exploitation and, possibly, violence.

As opposed to this perspective, abuse-oriented therapy assumes what to many is intuitively obvious: Children have less power than adults, are dependent on them, and are intellectually incapable of free and informed consent to have sex with them (Finkelhor, 1979b). This position must be nonnegotiable for the therapist. Further, I would argue that it is incorrect to assume that children inherently desire *sexual* contact with adults in the first place. They do, however, have needs for nurturance, love, contact comfort, and other affectionate expressions. Finally, even in those relatively uncommon instance where a child behaves in a truly seductive manner, as may occur when she or he has already been sexualized by previous molestation experiences (Friedrich, 1994), the adult's moral (and legal) obligation to resist such approaches is transcendent.

What does this issue mean for work with adult sexual abuse survivors? The victim of an assault or crime is more likely to feel rapport with and support from a therapist who sees her as an injured party, as opposed to a guilty coconspirator. As indicated in previous chapters, the survivor is often plagued by feelings of guilt and responsibility—reactions that should be ameliorated, not reinforced. Additionally, certain healing processes in abuse-oriented therapy, such as the healthy expression of anger and other aspects of working through trauma, require that the survivor understand the extent of her injury at the time and the coping strategies she necessarily marshaled to survive—psychologically or otherwise. Such therapeutic processes are unlikely in an atmosphere where the client is led to believe that either the abuse never happened, or, if it did, that it was his or her responsibility.

Phenomenological Perspective

A phenomenological perspective emphasizes the notions of reaction and accommodation in the development of later abuse-related problems, as described in chapters 1 and 3. It views many of the symptoms of postabuse trauma as logical, adaptive responses to victimization that become inappropriate in the postabuse environment, as conditioned reactions to abuse-related stimuli that persist into later life, or as seemingly dysfunctional behaviors that actually address painful internal states. This approach denies the need for convoluted concepts in the analysis of abuse-related psychological dysfunction, instead understanding such adult "pathology" as the psychological extension of early reactions and solutions to aversive childhood events.

As well as helping the therapist to understand the child's experience of abuse, a phenomenological analysis points to the need to "stay with" the client's experience in adulthood. Among other constraints, this perspective discourages the use of abstract interpretations or intellectualizations—even when such statements are technically true, let alone when they are based on experientially remote (e.g., Oedipal) concepts. Thus, for example, although statements like, "It sounds as if you feel out of control of your life, like when you lived with your mother" might be appropriate, the interpretation "I wonder if you aren't acting this way so I'll stop you from getting into trouble and thereby prove I care in ways that your mother never seemed to" is not. The latter statement, for example, assumes (a) that the client's behavior is "for" the therapist (although a possibility, nevertheless a relatively therapist-centered and client-negating comment); (b) that the client is in control of behaviors that, in fact, he or she may experience as compulsive or otherwise out of his or her control; (c) that the client may be symbolically or otherwise covertly requesting that the therapist assume control (something that may more accurately reflect the clinician's needs than the client's); and (d) that the client would ultimately construe such control behaviors as caring.

This injunction to stay with the client, rather than with a theory that may (or may not) fit her, applies not only to the content of therapist interventions but also to the process of treatment. Most important, the therapeutic ebb and flow must fit the client's (as opposed to therapist's) current psychological and emotional state, so that the content and process of therapy are congruent with the client's immediate experience and her ability to process new information or feelings. When therapist statements are "out of synch" with the client's present experience, they will be seen either as a disconfirmation of the client's reality (e.g., statements that "It's OK to feel angry" when the client is, in actuality, in a state of mourning—a mismatch that may cause the survivor to believe he or she *should* feel differently), or as evidence that the clinician, like many others, does not understand him or her. Although both of these concerns are relevant to work with most clients, the sexual abuse survivor, as described earlier, is especially vulnerable to feelings of "wrongness" ("I'm not feeling/thinking the right things") or social isolation ("My therapist doesn't understand either").

Finally, the survivor's internal state must be continually evaluated regarding the pace of therapy. As noted in chapter 6, a common danger in this regard is the clinician's tendency to move faster than the survivor is able to follow. This desynchrony may be due to the fact that although the therapist is "hot on the trail" of meaningful connections and insights, the client is having to confront and experience frightening memories, images, and affects—a process for which he or she may feel unprepared. Faced with what appears to the therapist as a sudden unwillingness to deal with certain abuse issues, the clinician may assume that resistance has set in and interpret this conclusion to the client. Although the concept of resistance has some validity in work with abuse survivors, behaviors that appear to be resistance may be, instead, the client's appropriate attempts to titrate (adjust the emotional intensity of) the therapeutic process. Such adjustments allow the survivor to digest new ideas or discoveries at her own rate, as well as ensuring her continued control over the psychotherapy session.

In its milder forms, this titration may involve periods of silence, dissociation, not understanding certain (manifestly understandable) points or concepts, or sudden changes in the direction of discussion. At more extreme levels, this attempt to slow or stop the rapid rate of painful clinician-induced affects may include "acting out"; verbal attacks on the therapist; attempts to distract with sexualized material; a sudden increase in adversariality; or, in the worst case, abrupt termination of therapy. Such client behaviors appear to be, at their roots, further survival behaviors—invoked against currently perceived dangers as opposed to childhood ones. Perhaps the key notion here is that the client generally knows best; assuming that she is invested in therapy, she will generally move almost as fast as her internal processes will allow. In this context, so-called resistance is often a message to the therapist to adjust the intensity or speed of his or her interventions downward.

Interestingly, respect for the client's need to regulate the flow of therapy does not preclude certain forms of confrontation by the therapist—especially vis-à-vis client distortion of the therapeutic relationship or his unnecessary use of defenses so primitive that they render treatment ineffective. Although this issue is covered in a later chapter, it is noted in passing that the experienced therapist should be able to discriminate between appropriate client reactions to process errors (feedback) as opposed to specific attempts by the client, based on an underestimation of her own strengths, to reduce anxiety by derailing effective psychotherapy (true resistance).

Egalitarianism

By definition, sexual abuse occurs in a context of powerlessness, intrusion, and authoritarianism. Because therapy for sexual abuse trauma is intended to remedy the effects of such dynamics, it is important that the treatment process not recapitulate them. Experience suggests, in fact, that authoritarian, power-laden interventions are likely to result in a variety of negative survivor behaviors, such as manipulation, rage, or "acting out," or in attempts by the client to produce therapeutic material that will please the therapist.

In his or her most obvious form, the authoritarian therapist presents as the all-knowing expert who tells the client what her problem is (sometimes including what her "repressed" childhood history consists of), how she is feeling about it, and what must be done to fix it. A more sophisticated version of this type of clinician is also common: Implying by her behaviors that she is certain of who the client is and what he needs, this therapist often projects the frustrating message "I know, but I won't tell." In either incarnation, such therapists are often distant beings who, at best, are most comfortable interacting in the mode of the benevolent parent or wise authority figure. Because they are the expert, any setbacks or problems that occur must be the client's fault, or a result of the client's pathology or resistance to treatment. Interestingly, such clinicians are often highly invested in analyzing a specific notion of "transference," whereby any negative reaction the client has to the therapist is interpreted as the client's long-standing issues with parental figures. Unfortunately, it is possible that the survivor's reactions to such therapists are precisely because the clinician *is* acting as a harsh parent or abuser (Elliott & Briere, 1995). In such an environment the survivor is also likely to experience transference associated with unresolved abuse issues because the current therapy setting actively recapitulates them.

For an example of the potential hazards of authoritarian interventions, consider the frequent correlation between such behaviors and subsequent client "acting out." What is the client to think if (a) the therapist is an expert who, by his behavior, implies omnipotence, but (b) the client continues to feel considerable emotional pain? It must be that the therapist is withholding the cure from the client because he has the power to bestow it. If so, then either (a) the therapist does not like the client, and is intentionally hurting him (as did his abuser in times past); or (b) the therapist is insensitive and does not know how bad the client is feeling (as may have been true of others in the survivor's early history). In the former instance, the survivor's rage is often restimulated, and a variety of retaliatory behaviors may ensue. In the latter case, the survivor may feel that he has to show the clinician just how disturbed or dysfunctional he really is through suicidal threats, increasingly disorganized behaviors, or more florid clinical presentations during the therapy session. As a result of this perceived betrayal (a major issue for many survivors), the therapist may undergo the oft-cited transition from idealized savior to devalued villain.

A second version of the authoritarian therapist is one who informs the client of his or her abuse history (regardless of the client's disclosure or lack thereof), and definitively ascribes all difficulties that she might experience to this history. Any client objection to this analysis may be interpreted as "denial" or "repression," and multiple interpretations may be made in the service of getting the client to see the "true" basis of her concerns. This version of controlling behavior may not be as obvious to some, because it appears to support an abuse perspective. Rather than being survivor-supportive, however, it is implicitly authoritarian and often destructive because it assumes that the therapist knows and the client does not. Ultimately, this therapeutic approach no more respects client autonomy and dignity than does the more classic authoritarian style.

As opposed to such perspectives, good abuse-focused therapy is most successful when it fosters a relatively egalitarian atmosphere, whereby the client is seen as a partner in treatment (Enns et al., 1995). Although this approach does not discount the experience, training, and skills of the therapist (nor the power imbalance entailed in any helper-helpee relationship—especially a funded one), it nevertheless assumes that, ultimately, the client is the authority regarding what transpired in his or her childhood, what postabuse trauma feels like, what seems to help and what does not, and whether therapy is progressing as it should. It further assumes that therapists are human beings who inevitably make mistakes and who may not always be able to maintain the empathic bond that guides accurate helping behaviors. Finally, more egalitarian therapy fosters independence in the client; both specifically from the therapist, and more generally in terms of his or her own individuation from powerful others.

From this perspective, "cure by the therapist" is replaced with "recovery by the survivor" with assistance from the therapist. This redefinition is not mere rhetoric. Ideally, the client is made aware early in treatment that good therapy is more an environment than an inherently curative procedure; assuming that the clinician can provide a safe, healing context, and helpful guidance, the client is in charge of her own recovery process.

Growth and Strength as Operating Assumptions

Like several other therapies, the philosophy of treatment advocated here for sexual abuse survivors stresses a growth model rather than a clinical one. The survivor is not seen as inherently "sick" but, instead, as someone who has made situationally appropriate accommodations to a toxic environment. These accommodations were healthy at the time of the abuse, and thus the client's current task is more one of learning new skills (both internal and external), updating survival behaviors and perceptions, and desensitizing traumatic stress than it is being cured of an illness. Unfortunately, the abuse environment may have been so insidious, chronic, and grievous that these learned responses were, to some extent, "burned in" or overlearned so that new, seemingly contradictory, learning is often difficult. In addition, by the time the typical abuse survivor is able to access therapy, he or she has already spent a number of years evolving a life view and an ingrained way of dealing with the world, the bulk of which was directly or indirectly affected by his abuse experiences.

For this reason, the learning of new perspectives, skills, and associations is a long-term endeavor, both in and out of therapy. In fact, one is never cured of an abuse history; one can only process, desensitize, and integrate those experiences, slowly change one's relationship to the memories, and live more fully in the present. In this regard, the client should be warned that she will never not have been abused—the past will continue to exist as memories, and it will always be a part of her life. In many cases, the past need not, however, continue to be an acute and overwhelming source of adult symptoms and discontent.

In eschewing a pathology perspective and stressing the adaptive basis of postabuse difficulties, abuse-centered therapy reveals itself to be less interested in client weaknesses than client strengths and capacities. In fact, the term *abuse survivor* emphasizes the fact that the victim persevered despite his or her psychic injuries. In the words of one psychotherapist: "I keep forgetting what she's been through. I think I know what happened, but it's harder to realize that she made it through it all. I'm honestly not sure I could have." As later chapters describe, this resilience and willingness to struggle should be reinforced and relied on by the therapist, whose task is lessened by the existence of the "strong, healthy part" in most survivors.

Context of a Victimizing Culture

Although many clinicians see psychological difficulties as primarily intrapsychic events, studies in areas as diverse as psychological anthropology, sociology, and community psychology stress the impact of an individual's culture on his or her mental health. Perhaps nowhere is this cultural contribution more obvious than in therapy with victims of socially prevalent acts of violence. As noted in the introduction, in our culture about one fourth to one third of women and one fifth to one sixth of men have experienced some form of sexual molestation as children. These numbers suggest that sexual abuse is, to some extent, a socially supported (or at least not socially prevented) phenomenon, much in the way as has been demonstrated for rape (Brownmiller, 1975; Burt, 1980; Koss & Harvey, 1991; Malamuth, 1981; Malamuth & Briere, 1986) and wife battering (Bograd, 1984; Walker, 1979). This *exteropsychic* aspect of sexual victimization has ramifications for the survivor that should be addressed in therapy.

The cultural aspects of the survivor's victimization are, at minimum, fourfold: (a) adversarial social forces that support the devaluation and exploitation of those with lesser social power (especially women, children, and the aged—each of whom are common targets for abuse and exploitation in North America); (b) cultural dynamics that seek to deny or discount the results of such victimization, by referring to valid abuse disclosures as lies, distortions, or false memories, or by blaming the abuse on the victim; (c) social reactions to the abuse survivor's subsequent behavior, based on his or her inferred abnormality and deviation from social norms regarding what is appropriate conduct; and (d) socialization of the psychotherapist, such that he or she, too, is prey to aspects (a) through (c) and thus may be less able to assist optimally the survivor in the process of recovery.

The therapeutic implications of the first three social aspects are substantial. Perhaps most important, and as noted in chapter 3, the survivor is frequently driven to construct meaning from her abuse and thus may benefit from therapy that includes a didactic component. These information-providing functions of abuse-focused therapy ideally work to counter the former victim's socially learned assumptions regarding her victimization, such as the notion that she was responsible for what transpired, or that sexual victimization is a rare occurrence that happens only to abnormal individuals. Therapists who attempt to externalize survivors' self-blame by attributing all aspects of the abuse to the perpetrator alone run several risks. These include the client's continued sense of guilt by association (e.g., "OK, so we were *both* screwed up") and the likelihood that specific, idiosyncratic aspects of the abuse will be used by the survivor to explain away the abuser's culpability (e.g., "Well, he was drunk at the time," or "He was lonely").

Compared with a perpetrator-only perspective, a social analysis of sexual victimization may facilitate certain aspects of psychotherapy. Perhaps foremost of these, attempts to externalize the client's self-blame (and stigmatization by others) may be aided by her awareness of social factors, such as cultural attitudes supporting the exploitation of those with lesser social power, and the widespread sexualization of youth by the media that indirectly contributed to her abuse (Enns et al., 1995). The notions that "it happened because of what I did and who I am" or that "I am different (and worse) than everyone else because of what happened to me" may become less tenable when the survivor truly understands the extent of sexual exploitation and victimization of women and children in our society, and, in fact, its prevalence throughout recorded history. Such insights may lead to a healthy anger at "the system"—typically a considerable improvement over equivalent anger turned inward.

> Andrea, a 43-year-old woman, works as a secretary at an architectural firm. She has been married for 17 years to the same man and has three teenage sons. Sexually abused from ages 7 to 13 by an older brother, Andrea has experienced periods of severe depression and anxiety throughout much of her life. Until 3 years ago, her major recourse had been a heavy reliance on supportive psychotherapy, tranquilizers, and occasional trials of antidepressant medication, as prescribed by her psychiatrist of 11 years. Although these interventions provided some intermittent relief, they served to convince Andrea that she was "mentally ill" and that she would require medical care for the rest of her life.
>
> When Andrea's therapist retired, she began seeing a female psychiatrist, who insisted she gradually reduce her dependence on medication and encouraged her to attend a group for incest survivors. Unlike her previous psychiatrist, this therapist stressed the role of victimization in Andrea's chronic distress, suggested books on incest and women's issues, and continually highlighted the "negative trade-offs"

she had been trained to make in terms of giving to other (e.g., as a wife and mother) rather than caring for herself. Initially resistant to her therapist's self-described feminist analysis, Andrea eventually became excited about the notion that "the problems aren't all me." In the last 2 years of treatment, she has not experienced a major depressive episode, although her coworkers and family see her as generally more irritable and more difficult to get along with. Andrea, herself, is clear about her psychological status: "I'm getting stronger now and more mad than scared. And I'm still growing."

As important as its impact on the content of psychotherapy, a social analysis also highlights the potential for cultural forces to impact on the psychotherapist. If we assume that sexual abusers are, to some extent, socialized as such in our culture, then we must also accept the probability that these same social forces influence the clinician's perceptions and behaviors as well. Such social training may cause the therapist to deny instances of sexual victimization when confronted with them, blame the victim for his or her molestation when abuse cannot be denied, and discount abuse effects when victimization as been established. Such social biases occur at many levels and in many individuals, including well-meaning experts in child abuse. Thus, the issue is less one of blaming clinicians whose attitudes are potentially destructive than of confronting the socially ingrained assumptions that reside within us all and that may creep into therapy when we least want or expect them to.

SUMMARY

This chapter has outlined some of the major philosophical issues involved in therapy with adults who were sexually molested as children. Overall, it is suggested that optimal work with sexual abuse survivors demands respect and acceptance of the client's personal experience and encourages awareness, growth, emotional processing, and skill development. The following chapters include several additional recommendations regarding the therapist's orientation to practice with abuse survivors. These suggestions, however, will be more directly integrated with specific techniques or discussion of specific clinical problems.

Vagaries of the Therapeutic Relationship: Transference and Countertransference

5

As important as are the specific abuse-focused treatment techniques and activities outlined in subsequent chapters, at least as crucial is the quality of the therapeutic relationship per se. Psychotherapy is, ultimately, a highly personal interaction between two people—each of whom is unavoidably the product of a long chain of life experiences. Thus, although we may sometimes wish to see therapy as a corrective procedure or entirely objective clinical intervention, it is more accurately understood as a special form of human relationship. As with other types of relationships, both members of the psychotherapy dyad are vulnerable to biases in perception and expectation as they seek to define and understand one another. Abuse-specific treatment may be especially difficult in this regard because it directly accesses childhood trauma and thus increases the likelihood that current interpersonal behaviors will be affected by historical events.

When the distortions in perception and expectation occur in the client, we refer to therapeutic *transference*, whereas similar effects on the clinician are described as *countertransference*. Because of the critical importance of these processes, especially in terms of their ability

---

Parts of this chapter were adapted from Elliott and Briere (1995).

to derail or inform effective abuse-focused psychotherapy, each is considered in some detail subsequently. This chapter concerns itself primarily with transferential and countertransferential dynamics as they relate to individual psychotherapy. Such issues emergence in other modalities as well, however, including group (Abney, Yang, & Paulson, 1992) and family (Shay, 1992) therapies.

TRANSFERENCE

As used in this book, transference can be defined as contextually inappropriate perceptions and expectations of significant others in one's adult life—including one's therapist—based on important interpersonal learning that occurred in childhood. This definition is more inclusive than that of the traditional psychoanalytic perspective, which more often focuses on the projection of Oedipal or pre-Oedipal dynamics per se.

It may be useful to divide transference, broadly defined, into three overlapping domains: (a) those chronic distortions of adult interpersonal perception that reflect a general world view skewed by childhood experience, resulting in archaic responses to relevant interpersonal stimuli, including one's therapist; (b) responses associated with early childhood disruption of the child-caretaker attachment bond, restimulated by the authority and caretaking function of the therapist; and (c) more acute, dramatic emotionality that arises when some aspect of the survivor's current interpersonal environment (including therapy) restimulates childhood issues or traumas. A final form of biased (although technically not transferential) perception involves the effects of the survivor's sex-role training. This phenomenon is addressed in chapter 10.

Cognitive Distortions

Many of our most basic assumptions and beliefs about ourselves, others, and the future are developed during childhood. As a result, the adult survivor's perception of the therapist and the therapeutic relationship are often affected by her childhood reactions to maltreatment, and her attempts to make sense of the abuse. These cog-

nitions were initially logical, developing out of the victim's perception of herself as helpless and inadequate, and her environment as
inherently dangerous. In adulthood, these cognitive sequelae can
result in low self-worth, passivity, expectations of betrayal and continued victimization, and hypervigilence to danger. Such perspectives and expectations inevitably affect everyday relationships, let
alone the therapeutic one.

Not only does sexual abuse teach the survivor that others can be
dangerous, it alters his or her perceptions of and response to power,
intimacy, and relationship—all of which are present during psychotherapy. One effect of this process is the survivor's tendency to
project abuse-based understanding of powerful others onto the therapist. As a result, the clinician can become more of a representation
of what the client expects or fears (e.g., betrayal, rejection, or
exploitation) than a real person. This representation, in turn, motivates reactive and defensive behaviors during treatment that are less
relevant to the actual therapeutic situation than to events long past.

There are several distortions that can occur in the survivor's perception of the therapist. These include at least three common patterns: *perpetrator, rescuer,* and *lover.*

When the therapist is seen as *perpetrator,* he or she is viewed as
one who requires obedience and appeasement. Based on experience
with abusive or neglectful caretakers in the past, the survivor may
assume that her worth is predicated on her ability to satisfy the
needs and expectations of power figures. The client's resultant
desire to please can result in seemingly blanket acceptance of the
therapist's statements about, and recommendations for, the client.
By uncritically accepting this "good client" behavior, the therapist
may reinforce a related survivor's assumption—that independence
and self-efficacy in relationships with powerful others are virtually
impossible.

When the therapist is unable or unwilling to weaken the association between the power attributed to the clinician role and the survivor's assumptions of resultant danger, the client will continue to
project on the therapist abuser-like characteristics. In response to
these projections, the survivor may feel fear or anger, each of which
can motivate behaviors that were adaptive in, or reactive to, the
original abusive relationship. When fear is evoked, the survivor

may engage in acquiescence, placation, or grooming of the therapist, or avoidance responses to treatment. He or she may be especially fearful of exhibiting independence of thought or action, believing that the therapist demands dependence and fealty. In this way, the other-directedness of the survivor may be reinforced rather than ameliorated.

In contrast to fearful responses, transferential anger can result in what appears to be highly inappropriate expressions of rage during treatment. Among the qualities of therapy that can stimulate perpetrator transference are the closeness of the therapeutic relationship, the greater authority and power of the clinician, and the likelihood that the therapist and perpetrator share the same gender and relative age status. In addition, and somewhat ironically, both the therapist and the perpetrator intentionally intrude and impact on the survivor, although their actions and goals differ. When such transference is in effect, the survivor's anger may be easily triggered, even by implicitly benign therapist behaviors that nevertheless remind the former victim of her or his abuser. For example, the clinician's manner of speaking, dressing, or gesturing may evoke client irritability or even dissociated outbursts.

Other therapist activities, however, are more clearly inappropriate or ill advised, such as visible impatience, unnecessary interruptions, or the appearance of discounting the client's concerns—behaviors that can stimulate client "overreaction" by virtue of their similarity to more extreme abuser actions in the past. Finally, some therapist behaviors stimulate angry transferential responses because of, ironically, their positive nature. Caring, complimentary clinician behaviors, for example, may trigger survivor rage if, during her childhood, such activities were originally used by her abuser for entrapment or were engaged in to ensure or reward victim compliance. In addition, therapist supportiveness may engender anxiety and subsequent anger in the survivor because she, in fact, values and longs for such attention and thus has more to lose if the clinician abandons her.

Another client response to her power projections onto the therapist initially motivates idealization rather than obvious fear or anger. The client may fantasize the therapist as *rescuer*—the one who was longed for when the survivor was being abused as a child, the antithesis of the perpetrator role. The therapist is placed in the role of an all-knowing, all-powerful being, on whom the client is magically bestowed both protection and cure. As a result, the survivor may view her position as that of the recipient of the therapist's wisdom and healing powers. This projection often results in the client assuming a passive or receptive stance in therapy. Because the client believes she has found someone whose power will protect and magically heal, she can become less motivated to do things for herself, seeking instead to engineer the right conditions, demands, or prompts for the therapist's beneficence. Ultimately, this transference may result in survivor anger, as the inevitably human therapist violates the idealized role by failing to neutralize the client's pain, fill her emptiness, or maintain constantly accurate empathy. At such times, the therapist may become devalued into a perpetrator.

A final cognitive transference pattern involves the therapist as *lover*. Although the client's responses to his or her therapist sometimes include sexual thoughts, especially during intensive psychotherapy, this dynamic is intensified considerably if the client is a survivor of sexual abuse, and the therapist is of the same gender as was the original perpetrator. Sexual issues may become even more salient if the survivor was originally forced to participate in her abuse (e.g., trained to stimulate the perpetrator or to behave as if abuse were desirable), if no violence occurred, or if the molestation occurred over an extended period in the context of an ongoing relationship that had some positive elements.

Eroticized transferential interactions with the therapist may include flirtation, sexual suggestions or invitations, and dressing or acting in a manner intended to be sexually interesting or arousing. These behaviors are often stereotyped, however, as if the survivor were acting the role of a seductive person in a play. Prominent characteristics of such client behavior are the (frequently dissociated) intensity of the behavior and the extent of hypervigilance regarding its effect on the clinician.

Part of this transferential distortion may reflect sexual or romantic associations to power, developed when the exploitation and boundary violations of abuse were combined with positive attention, sexual feelings, or perpetrator statements of love. The survivor may come to feel that positive responses from powerful others are inherently sexual or romantic and that the acquisition of such power figures is a basis for happiness. Faced with this goal, the survivor may call on the lessons learned during sexual abuse: that access to his or her body and sexual repertoire are powerful motivators and that boundaries are made to be transgressed. The client may pursue special times with the therapist, request late evening sessions, or attempt to initiate late-night telephone contact. There may be a desire to be the therapist's "one and only," in a way that he or she assumes only sexual intimacy can confer. This need may become elaborate and a source of rich and frequent sexual fantasies, especially when the therapist is unable or unwilling to address this transference.

Lover transference is rarely equivalent to actual sexual interest, however. It often reflects the intrusion of sexually related issues into what are not inherently sexual interactions. For example, the client may interpret his therapist's caring responses as sexual, and, as a result, may respond with behaviors that he learned in childhood are indicated in the presence of an interested or attracted adult: a sexualized but not necessarily sexual response.

Even the more commonly assumed scenario—that of the client who behaves in an explicitly sexual manner—is often not sexually motivated per se, despite the many concerns voiced by clinicians regarding seductive patients. Instead, the survivor may be (a) making assumptions, based on early abuse experience, about what sorts of basically dissociated and stereotyped behaviors are expected of her by this powerful other; (b) seeking support, affiliation, and protection in the only way she knows; or (c) attempting to turn an anxiety-arousing situation into a more familiar one. In those relatively infrequent instances where actual sexual gratification appears to be the goal of the survivor's behavior during treatment, such desires frequently reflect the client's conditioned association between sexual arousal and (originally coexisting) subjugation (Briere, Smiljanich, & Henschel, 1994).

Transference Involving Attachment Issues

As noted earlier, many sexual abuse survivors were also psychologically neglected early in life—an unfortunate correlation because both sexual abuse and early neglect are associated with attachment problems (Alexander, 1992). Disruption of the child-caretaker attachment bond can easily lead to significant interpersonal difficulties later in life, especially those associated with impaired self-reference and unmet needs for nurturance, protection, and love. Individuals with significant attachment difficulties are likely to project self-issues and unresolved nurturance/protection needs onto the client-therapist relationship. Especially relevant is the tendency for more severely injured survivors to experience (a) compelling needs for reliability, safety, and emotional connection; and (b) when he or she perceives deficiencies in these areas during therapy, to respond with abuse-relevant negative affects and distancing behaviors.

Survivor transferential expectations of parental nurturance during psychotherapy undoubtably reflects the tendency for unresolved attachment needs to be restimulated in any relationship with a potential parental figure. As such, the therapist can expect some survivors to be inordinately demanding during treatment, as the client projects onto therapy her childhood-appropriate rights to consistent parental support and loving attention.

Unfortunately for the survivor, the episodic and time-limited nature of psychotherapy and the necessary constraints of the psychotherapeutic relationship (e.g., therapist-client boundaries) can easily restimulate feelings of abandonment and betrayal—reactions that first occurred during the survivor's childhood deprivation of caregiver love and support. Just as the abandoned or unloved child responded with anger, fear, and sadness (Bowlby, 1973), the adult survivor may respond to appropriate therapist distance or minor therapist errors in empathy and attunement with rage, despondence, or terror.

The seemingly primitive character of some restimulated attachment can be startling to the unprepared therapist, as can the survivor's growing "neediness" for surrogate parental support and succorance as therapy continues and parent-child attachment dynamics intensify. It is just this reexperiencing of unmet attachment needs, however, that may allow the survivor to address childhood deprivation issues long after the fact, thereby providing an opportunity for the resolution of early trauma that otherwise would be unavailable for treatment. This reworking of attachment issues requires considerable patience on the part of the therapist and client, and calls on the therapist's ability to resist any countertransferential need to parent, join the survivor in boundary violation, or flee the therapy relationship.

Restimulation of Abuse Trauma

Although many survivor responses in therapy reflect the projection of cognitive distortions and attachment-related needs onto the client-therapist relationship, some of her reactions during treatment arise more directly from posttraumatic restimulation. These can occur either as dissociated abuse-era affects or therapy-triggered abuse-specific flashbacks.

Typically, dissociated abuse restimulation occurs when the survivor's history is triggered by an abuse-relevant stimulus during treatment (e.g., perceived or real rejection, abandonment, or maltreatment) that is reminiscent of a specific instance of severe childhood abuse or abandonment. Because of its surface similarity to unresolved childhood abuse issues, this stimulus can induce abuse "reliving" experiences, including powerful, dissociated feelings of rage, terror, loathing, sexual arousal, or grief, directed toward the therapist, client, or both. These emotional reactions often appear to occur without reason or context, in that neither the client nor the therapist are aware of their less immediate precipitants, and the dissociated character of the response may blur its connection to a specific therapeutic incident.

Alternatively, and less commonly, the client may respond to the therapist in the context of an actual flashback. For example, during an otherwise ordinary session the therapist may inadvertently trigger a powerful reexperiencing of a childhood abuse event, resulting in the client's falling into a dissociative state, striking out at the therapist, or screaming in a repetitive, stereotyped, contextually inappropriate fashion. Although such activities can be frightening to client and therapist, they are the result of restimulated posttraumatic stress as opposed to being a psychotic episode or necessarily evidence of severe psychopathology.

Although not evidence of mental disorder per se, the presence of dissociated abuse-era affects or abuse-specific flashbacks during therapy does often signal the presence of major unresolved child-hood trauma, as opposed to the more common difficulties of less psychologically injured clients. Such intrusions into the therapy ses-sion are not always included in the typical discussion of transfer-ence, partially because trauma-focused therapy only recently has been elucidated, and partially because transference is often de-scribed in terms of less acutely intrusive or more classically psy-chodynamic phenomena. Nevertheless, posttraumatic transference involving dissociated states and therapy-triggered intrusive experi-ences is an important aspect of work with sexual abuse survivors, both in terms of its disruption of "here and now" awareness in treat-ment, and its stimulation of intense affects that may not have obvi-ous meaning in the context of contemporaneous therapeutic events.

CLINICAL RESPONSE TO TRANSFERENTIAL ISSUES

Psychotherapy, almost by definition, involves client interactions with a powerful, psychologically important person in an intimate context. In this environment, the survivor is easily reminded of sim-ilar relationship configurations and scenarios from his or her early life, and thus is prone to seeing the therapist as a potential parent, victimizer, or unwanted conduit to the past. Therein lies the "catch" for the survivor: To resolve psychic injuries sustained in one or more abusive childhood relationships, he or she must voluntarily enter into what is, in some ways, an equally threatening one as an adult. The trust and hope that the survivor is somehow able to bring to this new relationship is, nevertheless, almost always incomplete. Also present are those painful feelings, cognitions, and perceptual systems the client experienced in childhood and a ten-dency to use those behaviors he or she initially invoked to survive ongoing trauma.

Viewed from this perspective, transference is seen not as a ther-apy-based neurosis but rather as the logical extension of the client's childhood experience. It additionally follows from this perspective that (a) client responses to her therapist can provide valuable infor-mation to both members of the therapeutic partnership regarding the survivor's early relationships and her current response to important or psychologically similar others; and (b) transference provides an opportunity to reconsider and process important childhood issues and interactions as an adult, without violence and exploitation.

To the extent that abuse-related transference is present, the therapist has the opportunity to facilitate the resolution of issues that, but for the capacity of humans to reenact unintegrated traumatic experience, might otherwise be unavailable for treatment. Working within the context of abuse-related transference also allows the survivor to update abuse-related assumptions and perceptions within a nonabusive adult relationship. Finally, because transference is a powerful restimulator of abuse-era affects, cognitions, and sensory experiences (e.g., flashbacks), abuse-focused therapy can be a place where traumatic memories are processed and desensitized, and new behaviors (e.g., greater affect regulation skills) are acquired.

It is, therefore, important that the clinician not respond to transferential behaviors as if they were directed at him or her as an independently existing person but, instead, view them as samples of the survivor's understanding of herself and others. The therapist who, for example, responds to rageful behaviors from her client with angry or punitive behaviors of her own runs the risk of recapitulating the original abuse dynamic and thereby reinforcing the survivor's belief that his victimization-based assumptions are correct.

It is not uncommon for abuse survivors to vent transferential anger at their therapists, who then respond punitively, thereby restimulating greater client rage, resulting in even harsher clinician behaviors, and so on. This downward spiral may eventually end in a frighteningly close approximation of the client's childhood experience of psychological victimization. As noted in a paper by Waldinger (1987) on "Intensive Psychodynamic Therapy with Borderline Patients" (the reader may wish to substitute the words "survivor of severe abuse or neglect" for "borderline"):

> The therapist must be able to withstand the borderline patient's verbal assaults without either retaliating or withdrawing, so that the patient's hostility toward the therapist is not buried but examined and understood as part of a more general pattern of relating to important others. (p. 268)

The need to view transferential anger not only as input regarding the survivor's sense of self and others but also as a chance to impact more positively on what otherwise might be another abuse scenario is noted well by Summit (1987), who states that

> the most minor failings from the therapist can trigger torrents of misplaced fury and fledgling righteousness. The need to either apologize or to punish ignores the meaning of the primary betrayal. While the client has every right to enrage or provoke, the therapist must attenuate angry or hurt reactions into supportive, optimistic responses. (p. 7)

It is not only angry transference that must not be reciprocated. As noted later in this chapter under "Countertransference," a few clinicians (most typically male ones; see, for example, Holroyd & Brodsky [1977], and Pope [1994]) are prone to sexual behavior with their clients—a proclivity that may be intensified when the client has formed a sexual transference to the therapist. Not only is therapist-client sexual contact manifestly unethical, and throughout North America illegal, it may represent the ultimate recapitulation of the survivor's molestation history. From such revictimization, the client learns not only that sexual abuse is a chronic event and that she still cannot trust intimacy or a relationship, but also that her sexuality is the most (or perhaps only) value that she has for others—even in the supposed sanctity of the client-therapist relationship.

The outcomes described previously highlight the ambivalence of the "seductive" abuse survivor. Although manifestly striving to introduce sexuality into the therapeutic relationship, she or he almost never truly wishes it to occur. The message "Let's be sexual (please don't show me that sex is what you want)" to some extent reflects the underlying conflict for many chronically abused children: Sexual contact signals betrayal and pain, but also sometimes produces temporary "love" and support.

Given the distinct possibility of sexualized client behavior, clinicians working with survivors of severe abuse must be prepared to respond to such transference in ways that do not reinforce sexualization, but remain supportive and helpful. Such therapist responses are usually noteworthy for the presence of three activities: nonparticipation, boundary clarification, and reframing.

Nonparticipation refers to the conspicuous absence of therapist involvement in sexualized interactions during psychotherapy. This may be as basic as overlooking the client's "accidentally" disarrayed clothing or not laughing at a sexually explicit joke, or as complex as choosing not to encourage a client's presentation of a sexual issue at a specific point in time because of one's intuition that the topic has been raised to distract or to sexualize the treatment environment. The goal of such studied nonparticipation is the client's perception that sex, although an important issue worthy of therapeutic exploration, is not a useful "hook" or bargaining chip in his or her relationship with the clinician. It is my experience that those therapists most concerned about (or reportedly plagued with) "seductive clients" are often among those who consciously or unconsciously reward such behaviors with increased attention and reactivity.

There are times when clinician nonreinforcement is insufficient to deal with client sexualization. The client, for example, who directly propositions his therapist is unlikely to stop doing so merely because the clinician does not enter into a discussion of her or his sexual interests. Similarly, the sexualized survivor who believes that therapist nonresponse to her sexual suggestions or invitations "is just part of the game" may not fully understand the clinician's nonparticipation as not being negotiable. In such instances, the therapist must instead address the issue more directly: by clarifying the boundaries between client and clinician, and by reframing the client's behavior in terms of its underlying motivation.

Boundary clarification involves the therapist's reiteration of the nonnegotiable limits of psychotherapy, including the absolute inappropriateness of client-therapist sexual or romantic behavior. Such proscriptions need not be presented in a harsh or punitive manner, although threatened, inexperienced, or aroused clinicians can be prone to a lecturing style in this regard. Instead, the client is reminded of the importance of having a relationship that is neither exploitive nor adversarial, one whose parameters and functions are all aboveboard, and, therefore, more trustworthy and reliable.

Finally, sexualized client behavior often can be rendered unromantic and nonproductive by being analyzed carefully as to its etiology and ultimate purpose in the session. This analysis may be positive in the sense that it affirms the survival basis of such behaviors and their logic earlier in life. Thus, for example, continuing client flirtation in a given session may be reframed by the therapist as an expression of the importance of the therapeutic alliance to the survivor, and as a way for the client to communicate her need for reassurance, approval, and even self-determination. Such reframes are perhaps most effective when they (a) directly (yet sensitively) identify the sexualized behavior, (b) interpret it as a historically logical but currently inappropriate way of communicating other needs, and (c) focus attention on the underlying emotional or interpersonal issues that motivate such behavior. When done well, such therapist feedback may be received positively by the survivor because it implies both deeper understanding and an unwillingness to be derailed from the process of assisting the client in her recovery.

COUNTERTRANSFERENCE

Transferentially based survivor issues demand considerable effort and clarity on the part of the clinician. He or she not only must correctly respond to evocative or challenging behavior, but also must keep from reacting on a personal level—despite the potential for survivor dynamics to activate the therapist's own historical issues or socially learned biases. As noted in the next section, this task is rarely completely accomplished, although careful attention to one's own issues, needs, and socialization can usually eliminate the potentially destructive aspects of negative countertransference.

As opposed to client transference, countertransference is defined here as biased therapist behaviors and reactions that are based on unresolved childhood needs or issues, or childhood learning that results in inappropriate adult responses. The therapist, despite his or her training and professional demeanor, is electing to enter into an intense, probably long-term relationship with someone who may have significant issues with attachment, intimacy, defense, and relatedness, and whose disclosures or actions may stir up or echo unprocessed aspects of the clinician's early life. There are at least two major sources of negative therapist countertransference to abuse-focused psychotherapy: the therapist's own childhood experience of abuse, maltreatment, neglect, or parental authoritarianism; and issues related to therapist gender.

Therapist's Childhood History

Based on the incidence data reported earlier in this book, we might predict that about one quarter to one third of female therapists and perhaps 10% to 15% of male therapists have sexual abuse histories, and that much larger percentages of each have been physically or emotionally victimized in childhood. Recent evidence suggests, however, that psychotherapists are even more likely than others to have been maltreated as children (Elliott & Guy, 1993; Pope & Feldman-Summers, 1992). Further, parental behaviors not severe enough to be labeled as abusive, such as a generally authoritarian, punitive, or emotionally withholding child-rearing style, may lead the (later adult) therapist to respond to clients in a similar manner. As a result, it is probable that childhood issues have personal relevance for many clinicians.

The impact of one's own history on working with survivors varies from person to person and from one situation to the next. On the one hand, if one's negative childhood history has been worked through in one's own therapy or in some other manner such that one's responses are integrated and relatively conscious, the experience of having "been there" can be a definite asset in working with survivors (Elliott & Briere, 1994). As a survivor himself, the therapist is likely to have a basic and sympathetic understanding of the client's dynamics, as well as a sense that positive outcomes are possible. Conversely, individuals who are still at odds with their childhood histories, who use denial, dissociation, or other avoidance defenses to deal with abuse-related dysphoria, are likely to discover that working with other people's victimization issues restimulates their own. This restimulation, in turn, usually increases the problems described in chapter 11, such as PTSD symptoms, dysphoria, and overinvestment or underinvestment in the client.

Classical Projection

Perhaps most typical of the intrusion of the therapist's unprocessed or unresolved childhood issues into his or her treatment of

survivors is the problem of projection. Specifically, because his negative childhood experiences or training may still be alive and well,
although often split off from consciousness, they can be activated by
the client's disclosures. This process may lead the therapist to project, misperceive, or misattribute her or his own difficulties onto the
client's. Thus, for example, the unconsciously angry therapist may
interpret client behaviors as rageful when, in fact, they more accurately reflect sorrow or may push the client to confront her abuser
when her strongest desire is actually to escape him. Similarly, the
fearful therapist with an unresolved history of psychological or
physical maltreatment may counsel the client to be careful, to watch
out, to be constantly vigilant for danger, or to forego challenging
experiences. In addition, the therapist raised by an autocratic, dom-
ineering father may respond to appropriate client challenges or
fledgling attempts at disagreement with authority as if they were
personal attacks or allegations of incompetence.

On a milder level, the therapist may project impatience or boredom
onto the client when, in fact, the therapist is the one having difficulties
with the pace or process of therapy. The therapist who has an excessive
need for control, perhaps based on childhood-related needs for safety
and predictability, may perceive the client as highly manipulative. The
clinician who has unresolved sexual issues may respond to innocuous
client behaviors as evidence that the client is being seductive.

Projection can be especially problematic because the survivor
inherently relies on the therapist for objective data and uncontami-
nated responses. The therapist must be able to assess the client's
state accurately to provide relevant therapeutic interventions. To the
extent that the therapist's past life events impairs his or her ability
to do these things, the client's progress in treatment is likely to suffer. Although the therapist who has worked through childhood
issues may have additional, helpful understanding of the client's
issues, the therapist who has not addressed early traumas may confuse his own history and needs with those of the client and, thus,
may be less able to provide accurate assessment and intervention.

Boundary Violation

Another major form of abuse-related countertransferential response is boundary violation. Any therapist behavior that intrudes

uninvited on the client, or violates his or her rights to self-definition can have the doubly negative effects of destroying the trust within which most important therapeutic work occurs, as well as directly discouraging the development of appropriate self-other demarcations. Such boundary violation includes any type of sexual behavior with clients, inappropriate personal disclosures, excessively intrusive questions or statements, habitual interruptions, violations of personal space, and the conscious or unconscious use of the client to gratify the therapist's needs.

Boundary violations may not always be recognized as such by the therapist, or may be seen as out of his or her control. These countertransferential boundary incursions typically arise from one of two phenomena: (a) the therapist's incomplete awareness of client-therapist boundaries because of his own inadequate boundary learning, or (b) as a form of reenactment of the therapist's childhood boundary violations. Neither of these dynamics reflects adequate psychological health in the psychotherapist, although, less major boundary distortions may not be as prognostically dismal as more major violations.

Depending on the extent of violation involved, boundary confusion can range from nontherapeutic to destructive. At minimum, such behaviors restimulate and reinforce abuse-related issues and trauma in the client, and potentially prevent or destroy the development of trust in the therapeutic relationship. At the most extreme end of the violation continuum, sexual abuse survivors are more likely than others to be sexually victimized by their therapists, and to suffer compounded distress and symptomatology as a result (DeYoung, 1981; Kluft, 1990; Magana, 1990; Pope & Bouhoutsos, 1986). Victims of less obvious therapist boundary violations (such as repeated exposure to intrusive questions, inappropriate statements, or lack of respect for client defenses) may suffer as well, either by way of a resurgence in postabuse trauma or by being deprived of a safe therapeutic environment.

Abuse survivors who have become therapists in an attempt to understand or resolve their own issues may find that they are, instead, overwhelmed by the needs and problems of survivor clients. As a result, psychotherapy may become chaotic, and boundaries between therapist and client may blur or dissolve. Less dramatically, the therapist may come to rely on the client for validation and support, such that the client's anger at the therapist or slow rate of recovery is seen by the clinician as a personal attack or invalidation. Because the client survivor is likely to have had many years of experience with role reversal and boundary violations, she may have little sense that such situations are inappropriate. In instances in which her projected anger toward the therapist evokes inappropriate therapist anger in return, she may ultimately perceive the therapy environment as verification of the continuing need for adversariality in adult relationships.

Avoidance

A final form of abuse-related countertransference is that which results in therapist dissociation and denial. Because the avoiding therapist spends considerable psychic energy keeping her abuse (or full realization of its meaning and impact) out of consciousness and his anxiety down to manageable levels, she may unconsciously work to prevent the client from exploring his own memories and feelings. In such instances, the clinician may actually become resentful of the client for restimulating her avoided memories or affects, and may present to her supervisor or consultant with complaints of client malevolence, hysteria, or self-indulgence.

Therapists can also feel emotionally overwhelmed by the amount of injury and distress to which they are exposed on a daily basis. This sense of being inundated by pain may be exacerbated by the therapist's own unresolved distress or trauma. Although some clinicians in this position overidentify with the presumed source of the pain (the client), others respond by emotionally distancing themselves from that source. The result is *underidentification*, although this term is a misnomer to the extent that the therapist is, in fact, being restimulated by the survivor.

The primary manifestations of underidentification are (a) cognitive attempts to minimize the pain and consequences of one's own child abuse by avoiding discussion of the client's abuse history, and (b) a generally decreased therapeutic attunement to the survivor client. In each instance, the underlying, usually unconscious strategy is the same: reduced contact as a way to reduce restimulated pain.

In the former case, therapist resistance to believing the survivor's child abuse history—and the psychic implications of that history—serves a psychological need, although it is rarely acknowledged as such by the clinician. The therapist may overrely on simplistic assumptions regarding the incidence or impacts of sexual abuse, primarily in terms of denying the existence or primacy of such maltreatment in the client's history. Although clients' abuse reports require the same level of clinical evaluation as do any other statements that occur during therapy, some clinicians become especially critical and disbelieving when abuse emerges as an issue during treatment. In any given instance, the therapist may be expressing appropriate concerns about the validity of a specific historical statement. It is likely, however, that some therapists who consistently reject abuse reports as fiction are motivated by the need to either (a) avoid restimulation of their own abuse-related issues and distress, or (b) circumvent the intrusion of their own sexual responses to the idea or images of their client involved in sexual (albeit forced) contact. By denying the reality, relevance, or importance of the client's childhood abuse history, the underidentified clinician may seek to apply the same rule to his or her own childhood pain or current sexual conflicts.

In contrast to complete rejection of the reality of abuse, another form of avoidance manifests as reduced attention or attunement to the client when abuse issues are being processed in therapy. When this presents as a chronic pattern, the clinician characteristically responds with relative indifference or professional coolness to the pain of survivors. Although professional objectivity is a necessary tool in the day-to-day management of what otherwise might be overwhelming work-related distress, its overdevelopment and over-application usually signals a more personal defense, frequently against one's own restimulated posttraumatic distress.

Some therapists, although generally able to interact with compassion during general clinical work, can enter a somewhat dissociated disattunement when upsetting abuse-related issues emerge during treatment. Unfortunately, such self-protective attempts to disengage from restimulating therapeutic events are frequently perceived by the client as disinterest or abandonment, thereupon triggering in the client the various transferential behaviors outlined earlier. This response, in turn, may further restimulate the therapist's countertransference, leading to reciprocating (and sometimes intensifying) transference-countertransference cycles and further derailing the treatment environment.

Gender-Related Issues

Therapist reactions to survivors also may be affected by their gender-specific childhood training. Although not strictly a countertransferential process per se, in the sense of representing the biasing effects of personal history, the lessons of a sexist or sex-role stereotypic society are nevertheless learned early in life and commonly distort subsequent interpersonal perception and expectation. Males in our culture, for example, are often socialized in adolescence by peers and role models to view most emotionally intimate relationships as potentially sexual ones (Finkelhor, 1984), resulting in a tendency to respond to certain essentially nonsexual interactions as if they were sexual in nature. Given this proclivity, male therapists must somehow unlearn this false equation early in their clinical careers if they wish to relate in nonpredatory ways toward women. Not all male therapists have done this, however, and thus some are prone to sexualizing female clients during psychotherapy.

This sexualization dynamic may be intensified in the presence of the female abuse survivor, whose frequent neediness and tendency to respond to male power with acquiescence or pseudosexual behaviors may make her a target for various forms of revictimization during treatment. Even those instances in which such therapists do not behave in an overly sexual manner, their overattention to the sexual aspects of the survivor's presentation (e.g., her attractiveness, anatomy, or disclosures regarding sexual issues) can alter the agenda from healing to adversariality and further harm.

Because of this potential for revictimization, several writers suggest that female abuse survivors should be seen only by female therapists. I generally agree with this principle and recommend that women survivors (especially those with more severe histories who were abused by a man) see women in therapy if an effective female therapist is available or, in any event, if the client requests one. It is not my experience, however, that all male therapists demonstrably sexualize their female clients, just as not all female psychotherapists are effective in the treatment of sexual abuse trauma in females. Some women who were sexually (or otherwise) abused by their mothers or other women may also feel considerably safer when working with a male therapist. Thus, in the absence of an available, qualified female clinician, or where the primary perpetrator was a woman, male-female therapeutic dyads may be acceptable or indicated. The issue then becomes one of determining which male therapists are appropriate for which female abuse survivors and, more globally, how the effects of male socialization can be ameliorated so that such screening is no longer necessary. The latter task is a long-term one, requiring changes not only in society as a whole but also specifically in the clinical training programs that produce psychotherapists.

The potential gender effects on female therapists, although more benign in terms of sexualization, can still be significant. The most frequent impact is probably overidentification. The therapist may closely relate to her female client's experience of victimization, based on her own history of being the target of male aggression, or her fears of such aggression. For example, it is probably far different for a male therapist to hear of a rape of a 13-year-old girl than it is for a woman to do so. The man, although perhaps empathic and sensitive, can understand the act of rape only intellectually unless he was, in fact, raped or feared raped himself at some point. The female therapist, conversely, has had a significant chance in her lifetime of being a victim of rape or attempted rape (Russell, 1983a), is likely to have feared the possibility of sexual assault since childhood or early adolescence, and may additionally fear the molestation of her own children in ways that differ from those of their father.

It should be noted at this point, however, that although these issues are more prevalent in one sex than the other, each may easily cross over to the other. Some female therapists sexualize their clients, and some formerly abused male therapists overidentify with the pain of their survivor clients. Further, although a therapist's childhood history and gender training have the potential to distort his or her therapeutic practice, such intrusion is probably not the rule in everyday therapeutic practice.

Intervention in Therapist Countertransference

Because of the critical importance of clinical objectivity and trust-worthiness in work with sexual abuse survivors, as noted earlier, unresolved countertransference must be addressed whenever (and, it is hoped, before) it intrudes into the treatment environment. Not only does countertransference affect the therapy and potentially derail effective treatment, it also signals therapist distress and the need for external assistance or intervention.

For these reasons, regular consultation is recommended as an important component of abuse-focused psychotherapy. Such structured support allows therapists to share the burden of daily exposure to others' pain, as well as to explore ways in which his or her own issues can distort perception and practice, producing negative therapeutic outcomes. In many instances, inappropriate identification or projection can be prevented or remediated by the consistent availability of an objective consultant who is alert to countertransferential issues in general, and the clinician's vulnerabilities in specific. Although minor overidentification or underidentification and projection often can respond to clinical vigilance alone, higher levels of these problems and almost any form of boundary confusion typically require outside intervention.

Because countertransferential issues especially prevent some therapists from acknowledging the reality and consequences of sexual abuse in their clients' lives, it is unlikely that such individuals will be helpful in resolving abuse-related trauma. Such clinicians should consider referring the client to a therapist experienced in abuse-focused psychotherapy, particularly when sexual abuse is the presenting problem.

Alternatively, for clinicians who acknowledge the impact of childhood issues in their own lives, psychotherapy may help address the intrapsychic etiology of the countertransference. It is likely, in fact, that some proportion of survivor-therapists require their own psychotherapy before they can work effectively with other abuse survivors. For such individuals, one's own therapy not only reduces abuse-related difficulties but also can result in an extraordinary psychotherapist— one who has directly experienced (and thus has a greater appreciation of) both childhood injury, and adult resolution and growth.

Boundary violations involving any sexual behavior or other major client exploitation—whether countertransferential or not—is of sufficient gravity that it requires immediate and incisive intervention (Pope, 1994). In the case of sexual contact with clients, the individual must remove himself or herself from the practice of psychotherapy, refer his or her clients to another therapist, and notify the appropriate professional and legal authorities. Less obvious boundary confusion may require less extreme actions; nevertheless, the therapist should seek objective consultation from another professional to determine the extent of the problem and the most appropriate interventions.

CONCLUSION: THE THERAPEUTIC RELATIONSHIP REVISITED

As described in this chapter, there are several potential barriers to effective abuse-focused psychotherapy, primarily associated with the psychological power of childhood history to affect both clinician and client. Additionally, as noted in chapter 4, treatment for the effects of abuse occurs within the same social matrix in which the original victimization took place, and thus the treatment process may be compromised by equivalent social dynamics. These various impediments need not necessarily derail effective psychotherapy, however, if the client's projection of early issues and training onto therapy is not overwhelmingly intrusive, if treatment boundaries can be maintained, and if the clinician is sufficiently aware of (and able to regulate) her or his personal issues and biases.

As noted earlier, the process of transference—when handled appropriately—can significantly enrich the treatment process by encouraging the client to confront and process abuse-based issues in the relative safety and supportiveness of the therapy session. Thus, the survivor in effective psychotherapy may (a) initially have unduly negative abuse-related expectations and understandings of therapy and the therapist, which (b) slowly give way to more positive and accurate perceptions as treatment progresses, and these assumptions are gradually seen to be inconsistent with the clinician's caring and trustworthiness, leading to (c) new learning about the potential for significant others to be benign and nonexploitive, despite what may be their surface similarities to the original abuser. This process is far superior to merely being *told* that not all powerful or personally important people are dangerous because it allows the survivor to experience this fact in vivo.

The ultimate repercussions of such transferential learning include decreased difficulties with authority, greater trust in relationships, a clearer sense of interpersonal boundaries, and the development of affiliative (rather than solely defensive or adversarial) social skills. Perhaps as important as any other therapeutic lesson, successful resolution of negative transference teaches the survivor that his or her abuse—as heinous as it may have been—is a historical event, not an inevitable outcome for present or future relationships.

Specific Therapy Principles and Techniques

6

This chapter introduces several specific principles and approaches that my colleagues and I have found useful in working with sexual abuse survivors. The interested reader is referred to other clinical texts or papers for additional information on abuse-relevant therapy for adults (Classen, 1995; Courtois, 1988; Enns et al., 1995; Meiselman, 1990; Olio & Cornell, 1993; Salter, 1995) and children (Berliner, in press; Friedrich, 1995, 1996; Lanktree, 1994) because any one source in this complex and rapidly growing area is likely to overlook important ideas and intervention approaches. Before the current methodology (described elsewhere as the Self-Trauma model [Briere, 1996]) is presented, however, a point arising from the material outlined in chapter 5 should be emphasized: No techniques can replace the respect and stable, affirming connection offered by good generic psychotherapy, irrespective of whether or not it is abuse oriented per se. There are many psychotherapists who, given attitudes and perspectives similar to those described in chapter 4, provide good treatment for abuse survivors without changing their usual therapeutic style. Thus, the interventions suggested by the current chapter should be seen as, for some readers, further sharp-

Parts of this chapter were adapted from Briere (1996), with the publisher's permission.

ening or focusing of what already may be effective therapeutic skills and approaches.

A corollary to this point is that use of these techniques will not necessarily make one a helpful therapist—one must already be able and prepared to listen, to support, and to confront gently when necessary, all the while remaining neither too close nor too distant. Many things aid in the development of such core therapist qualities, including effective clinical training, one's own therapy, experience in working with traumatized people, and the time and energy to introspect on "the meaning of it all." The latter point, as well as other aspects of being a therapist who works with survivors, is covered in detail in chapter 11.

TREATMENT PROCESS ISSUES

In light of these provisos, this chapter begins with a consideration of the process, rather than strictly content, of abuse-focused psychotherapy. Therapeutic process is concerned with the way in which treatment is conducted, and addresses issues such as how fast should treatment go with this client, when should the therapist explore new material, and when should the therapist focus on what. The notion of treatment process is explored subsequently in the context of what is described as the *therapeutic window.*

Phenomenology of Survivorhood

Appreciation of the importance of positive treatment process requires a brief return to the phenomenology of survivorhood outlined in previous chapters. Most basically, good therapy must acknowledge and honor the survivor's competing needs to maintain safety and internal stability while, at the same time, being open to information and experience so that he or she may heal and grow. Because, as outlined in chapter 3, many survivors of severe sexual abuse suffer from reduced self-resources, the survivor often finds herself balancing awareness of painful or threatening recollections and feelings with the need to avoid this same material so as to not be overwhelmed by it. Because many internal and external events have the potential to produce painful feelings or restimulate traumatic stress, this balance between engagement and safety can be precarious. The dilemma has been expressed by many survivors in treatment, often with some version of the following: "How can I open myself up [e.g., to treatment, relationships] if I don't know whether I will be hurt even more?"

The need to balance challenge with safety is perhaps never as obvious or relevant as during psychotherapy. On one hand, the client is often aware that she must confront painful material and try seemingly dangerous new behaviors to gain from treatment and move beyond her current state. On the other, she knows that she can be hurt by such activities if they exceed her internal capacities to accommodate them. For example, the client who allows himself to reexperience a childhood rape during treatment may either (a) slowly process and desensitize his painful responses to such memories and eventually develop greater control over his internal experience (as described later in this chapter); or (b) become overwhelmed by previously avoided revulsion and terror, with the result that he is flooded by flashbacks, intrusive memories, and seemingly uncontrollable panic. Because the client is intrinsically attuned to the risks of psychic exploration (or to greater immediate awareness of existing pain), he or she wisely approaches the therapeutic endeavor with caution and readily available defenses.

Therapeutic Window

Because the degree to which the client is able to tolerate abuse-related distress rests, in part, on the extent of his or her self-capacities, the clinician must keep both self- and trauma issues in mind when treating abuse survivors. He or she must carefully monitor and (to some extent) control the therapeutic process: facilitating access to painful material when the client can tolerate it, and avoiding or discouraging premature exposure to material when it has the potential to overwhelm, disrupt, or injure. It is in this context that we consider the *therapeutic window,* a concept somewhat similar to Olio's notion of the "affective edge" (Cornell & Olio, 1991; Olio & Cornell, 1993). The therapeutic window may be defined as the psychological "location" where effective psychotherapy for trauma inherently occurs: the place where (a) important therapeutic material is experienced and addressed, but (b) such material is introduced and managed in such a way that it does not overwhelm internal capacities, retraumatize, or foster excessive defensive avoidance in the session. From the therapist's perspective, the window represents the answer to the question: "How can I provide a therapeutic stimulus that moves the client beyond where she is, but that does not overwhelm her internal resources and produce excessive distress and further defense?"

Clearly, therapeutic interventions that are pitched short of the window or that exceed its outer limits are less effective and, in the latter instance, potentially harmful. Examples of undershooting the window are interventions that provide insufficient challenge or avoid important material. The clinician who steadfastly overlooks or discounts a survivor's child abuse history or whose focus is based solely on "supportive psychotherapy" (i.e., avoiding all psychological exploration) may not ever overwhelm the survivor, but he or she is also unlikely to provide significant assistance in the reduction of abuse-related difficulties. This is because effective therapy does not just support—it must on some level (a) evoke trauma-related memories, feelings, and thoughts so that they can be processed; (b) increase awareness; and (c) motivate the development of new responses. Because the survivor has learned to dissociate, anesthetize, deny, tension-reduce, and otherwise avoid in response to potentially threatening phenomena, he or she has a tendency to respond conservatively to therapeutic interactions. This sometimes means that the survivor will seek to maintain the status quo in treatment: seeking much-wanted support and nurturance from the therapist, but often avoiding affects or insights that upset and potentially overwhelm. In this context, the solely "client centered" or "supportive" psychotherapist—although rarely doing harm—is likely to accomplish only minor gains in the treatment of severe abuse trauma.

Conversely, therapeutic interventions that provide more stimulation or challenge than the survivor can accommodate run the real risk of being harmful. The survivor who has carefully reduced her awareness and extent of interpersonal functioning to match her underdeveloped self-reference and self-capacities will not benefit from interventions that topple this fragile balance. Examples of overwhelming interventions include (a) pushing the survivor to process material more quickly that is appropriate; (b) encouraging her or him to describe in detail that which requires further work or support before it can be safely discussed or processed; (c) exposing the client to overly stressful stimuli (e.g., inappropriately intensive role playing, group work, or guided imagery); (d) overly challenging or confronting statements or interpretations; (e) "uncovering" procedures (e.g., hypnosis) that expose the survivor to distressing material before she is strong enough to access them on her own; and (f) demands that the client "work harder" or "stop resisting" when, in fact, the client is titrating the intensity of the therapeutic environment correctly.

If a given therapeutic intervention does, in fact, exceed this balance, the survivor has little choice but to invoke defensive responses. These may include, at minimum, sudden therapeutic "resistance" (a misnomer for what is, in fact, usually reasonable attempts by the client to reduce the impact of therapeutic errors), avoidance of threatening topics, intellectualization, vagueness or mild dissociative disengagement, seductiveness, or argumentativeness over a peripheral issue. If the therapist's behavior is especially disruptive, the survivor may need to resort to more powerful dissociative activities or literal physical escape from the session. If these defensive responses are insufficient to restore equilibrium, the survivor may become increasingly symptomatic: He or she may experience repetitive flashbacks, extreme dissociative withdrawal, regression to more child-like states, or fragmentation of self-functioning. After a session in which his or her capacities were overwhelmed, there may be a need to engage in substance abuse or tension-reduction activities, such as self-mutilation or "compulsive" sexual behavior as a way to dampen excessive distress and return to equilibrium.

Fortunately, most therapy that misses the therapeutic window is less injurious than the preceding. More typically, the erring clinician does not completely avoid addressing every important issue, nor does he or she outrageously bombard the survivor with overwhelming material. Instead, ineffectual therapists tend to avoid more than is appropriate (often by virtue of social or countertransferential issues), or make errors in timing or empathy that threaten the survivor by indicating that the therapeutic session is not a safe or reliable place. In either instance, the net result is less than optimal treatment.

Given these concerns, how does one stay within the therapeutic window? Minimally, attention must be paid to two domains: assessment of the client's trauma level and self-capacities, and the process of providing balanced intervention.

Assessment

Because the concept of the therapeutic window inherently rests on assessment of the client's internal state, the clinician must be as aware as possible of both the survivor's current level of posttraumatic distress, and his or her immediate access to stabilizing self-capacities. This is best accomplished by formal psychological assessment at the onset of treatment and by ongoing attunement to the client's internal experience during therapy.

Regarding the former, the qualified clinician may choose to administer relevant psychological tests or refer the client to a psychologist who can provide this service. Although the clinician is directed to outside sources for a review of survivor-relevant testing approaches and assessment instruments (Briere, in press, a, b; Elliott, 1994b), several points should be made here. First, many standard psychological tests were developed without reference to the specific issues and difficulties associated with sexual abuse trauma, and therefore tend either to underevaluate abuse-related symptomatology or to overpathologize it. Second, those instruments currently available for the evaluation of psychological trauma often lack critical psychometric information on reliability, validity, and standardization, and tend to focus on a few symptom types (e.g., posttraumatic intrusion or avoidance).

In response to these potential problems, the assessment-qualified clinician may wish to use the Trauma Symptom Inventory (TSI; Briere, 1995b). This is a standardized instrument that yields three validity and 10 clinical scale scores thought to tap the range of abuse- and trauma-related difficulties, including posttraumatic stress, dissociation, sexual problems, altered mood, and difficulties associated with impaired access to self-capacities (see Appendix 1 for further information on this measure). The TSI or another multi-modal trauma instrument, in combination with appropriately interpreted data from tests such as the Rorschach, Minneosta Multiphasic Personality Inventory (MMPI)–2 (Butcher, Dahlstrom, Graham, Tellegen, & Kaemmer, 1989), or MCMI-III (Millon, 1994), can provide the clinician with considerable information on three aspects of the survivor's internal experience: his or her trauma symptoms, level of dysphoria, and access to stabilizing or regulating self-capacities. Knowledge of the first two, as balanced by the third, for example, may allow the clinician to determine the extent to which the survivor is potentially free to address new material or whether he or she is generally overwhelmed by abuse-related symptoms and dysphoria, and requires more basic support and less exposure to traumatic material.

Even more important than appropriate psychological testing, however, is the therapist's ongoing attunement to the client's internal experience. This is because (a) psychological test data are most relevant to the client's self-reported psychological state at the onset of treatment, as opposed to his or her psychological functioning at later points; (b) such testing is more concerned with enduring psychological features or traits (e.g., the general presence of posttraumatic stress or impaired self-reference), whereas the survivor's immediate experience may change rapidly within and between sessions; and (c) some information about the survivor's state and internal equilibrium often can be determined by only her or his response to therapist behaviors and the therapeutic relationship. Further complicating the assessment process is the possibility that fluctuating dissociative or denial-based defenses may lead the survivor to underreport distress or symptoms on psychological tests—a scenario often better recognized (and adjusted for) by the clinician during the psychotherapy session.[2]

Empathic attunement to the survivor's internal state often involves ongoing assessment of his or her relative balance between traumatic stress and self-capacities. The survivor who becomes ex-

---

[2]Although the TSI has validity scales that can identify the presence of this possibility, it is not easy to correct for such avoidance-related underreporting when it occurs.

cessively angry, anxious, despondent, or fragmented in response to careful therapist attempts to address potentially upsetting material, for example, may be revealing that she or he has insufficient self-capacities at the moment to tolerate much exposure to traumatic stimuli. Similarly, the client who reports flashbacks, nightmares, or excessive intrusive memories in response to prior therapeutic events may be signaling the need for less focus on potentially destabilizing material and more attention to the building of self-resources. Conversely, the survivor who is able to discuss potentially distressing experiences without overwhelming distress or the need to retreat to higher levels of dissociation, intellectualization, or denial is likely to have sufficient self-resources to permit further exploration and therapeutic processing.

Balanced intervention

At least three aspects of therapeutic process should be considered in effective abuse-focused psychotherapy. These are (a) exploration versus consolidation, (b) intensity control, and (c) goal sequence. Each reflects the therapist's attempt to find the appropriate point between support and opportunity for growth, with the assumption that, when in doubt, the former is always more important than the latter.

Exploration Versus Consolidation

This aspect of the therapeutic process occurs on a continuum, with one end anchored in interventions devoted to greater exploration and processing of potentially threatening (but therapeutically important) material, and the other involving interventions that inherently support and solidify previous progress, or that provide a secure base from which the survivor can operate without fear.

Exploratory interventions typically invite the client to examine or reexperience material related to his or her traumatic history. For some abuse survivors, exploration may involve not only development of insight but also a testing of the waters in the affective domain. For example, an exploratory intervention might involve asking the client to consider the possibility of using less cognitive avoidance or dissociation when describing a previously described painful subject. The key here is that the survivor—in the context of relative safety—attempts to do something new and potentially helpful, whether it is thinking of something previously not completely considered or feeling something previously not fully experienced.

Consolidation, conversely, is less concerned with growth than it is with safety. Consolidative interventions focus the client on potential imbalances between trauma and self at a given moment, and invite the client to shore up the latter. An important issue here is that the survivor is not being asked to avoid existing traumatic states, but rather to more fully anchor himself or herself in such a way as to strengthen faltering self-capacities. Interventions in this domain may entail, in one instance, grounding the agitated client in the "here and now." In another instance, it may involve reminding the client of how far he or she has come, and of the need to acknowledge his or her needs for safety.

The decision to explore or consolidate at any given moment reflects the therapist's assessment of which direction the client's balance between stresses and resources is tilting. The psychologically overwhelmed client, for example, typically requires less exploration and more consolidation, whereas the stable client may benefit most from the opposite. Further, this assessment of the client's internal state may vary from moment to moment: At one point exploration may be indicated, whereas at another consolidation may be required. From the therapeutic window perspective, exploration moves the client toward the outer edge of the window, where emotional processing and new insights may occur, whereas consolidation moves toward the inner edge, where safety is more predominant.

Intensity Control

Intensity control refers to the therapist's attempt to regulate the client's level of affect during the session. Most generally, it is recommended that therapeutic intensity be highest at around midsession, whereas the beginning and end of the session should be at the lowest intensity. At the onset of the session, the therapist should be respectful of the client's need to enter the therapeutic domain of trauma and self-work gradually, whereas by the end of the session the client should be sufficiently dearoused that she or he can reenter the outside world without difficulty. The relative safety of the session may encourage some clients to become more emotionally aroused than they normally would outside of the therapeutic environment. As a result, it is the therapist's responsibility to leave the client in as calm an affective state as is possible—ideally no more than the arousal level present initially—lest the client be left with more affective tension than he or she can tolerate.

Beyond the time-oriented aspects of intensity control, the therapist should appreciate what some have referred to as the survivor's dread of affect (Krystal, 1978). For those severely abused as children, there may be a fear that extreme anger will lead to violent behavior, and that extreme sadness will result in self-destructiveness. For others, immersion in abuse-related fear may seem to signal that childhood trauma is about to happen all over again (Krystal, 1978). Some survivors with major self-difficulties may unconsciously fear that extreme affect will engulf them or destroy their sanity. For such individuals, intensity control is a mandatory aspect of good therapy.

From the perspective offered in this chapter, intense affect during treatment may push the survivor toward the outer edge of the window, whereas less intensity will represent movement toward the inner (safer) edge. The need for the client, at some point, to feel seemingly dangerous feelings—not to dissociate or otherwise avoid them—during abuse-focused treatment requires that the therapist carefully titrate the level of affect the client experiences, at least to the extent this is under the therapist's control. The goal is for the client to neither feel too little (i.e., dissociate or cognitively avoid to the point that pain cannot be processed) nor feel too much (become so flooded with previously avoided affect that he or she overwhelms available self-resources).

Sequence of Therapeutic Goals

As noted by various authors (Courtois, 1991; Linehan, 1993; McCann & Pearlman, 1990), therapy for severe abuse-related difficulties should generally proceed in a stepwise fashion, with early therapeutic attention paid more to the development of internal resources and coping skills than to trauma per se. This principle considers the fact that those interventions most helpful in working through major traumatic stress may overwhelm the client who lacks sufficient self-resources (Linehan, 1993). Specifically, the process of remembering and desensitizing traumatic experiences requires basic levels of affect tolerance and regulation skills. In the relative absence of such self-resources, the processing of traumatic material can easily exceed the therapeutic window and lead to fragmentation, increased dissociation, and later involvement in tension-reduction activities—an outcome that is, sadly, not uncommon when the therapist is undertrained or inexperienced in trauma therapy.

As noted earlier, the choice of therapeutic goals for a client must rely on detailed psychological assessment. Unfortunately, because of the complex relationship between self-capacities and traumatic stress, assessment of readiness to do trauma work cannot be determined solely at one point and then assumed thereafter. Indeed, self-functioning may appear sufficient early in treatment, only to emerge as far less substantial later in therapy. For example, as therapy successfully reduces dissociative symptomatology, it may become clear that what originally appeared to be good affect regulation actually represents the effects of dissociative avoidance of painful affect. Alternatively, a client who initially had superficially intact self-functioning may later experience a reduction in self-capacities as he or she addresses especially traumatic material. Although some of this fragmentation may respond to careful therapeutic consolidation, it is also true that intense reexperiencing of traumatic events can temporarily reduce self-functioning (Linehan, 1993). Given these potential scenarios, it is strongly recommended that the therapist continue to evaluate the client's current self-functioning and trauma level throughout treatment, so that he or she can adjust the type, focus, or intensity of intervention when necessary.

Intervening in Impaired Self-Functioning

As described earlier, the availability and quality of self-resources are typically major determinants of the client's level of symptomatology, and his or her response to treatment. So important are self-resources to traumatic stress and therapeutic intervention that, as mentioned, some clients may require extensive "self-work" before any significant trauma-focused interventions can occur. For others, there may be sufficient self-skills available to allow some trauma-based interventions, yet continued attention to the development of further self-resources will be required. In relatively fewer clinical abuse survivors (usually those with less injurious early childhood experiences), self-issues may not require any significant intervention, and processing of traumatic material may occur more quickly (Linehan, 1993). Even in the latter case, however, it is possible for processing of especially painful traumatic memory to overwhelm normally sufficient self-capacities briefly, thereby requiring some (typically temporary) self-level interventions.

Safety and Support

For many survivors, the earliest hazard to the development of self-resources was the experience of danger, and lack of support or protection. As a result, these issues must receive continuing attention in abuse-focused psychotherapy. In the absence of continual and reliable safety and support during treatment, the survivor is unlikely to reduce her reliance on avoidance defenses, nor to attempt the necessary work of forming an open relationship with her therapist. Because early neglect or abuse may have led to the development of an ambivalent or avoidant attachment pattern (Alexander, 1992), the client is, in some sense, being asked to go against lifelong learning and become dangerously vulnerable to a powerful figure. That he or she is willing to do so at all in such cases is testament to the investment and bravery that many abuse survivors bring to therapy.

Given the preceding, the clinician must work hard to provide an environment where the survivor can "let in" therapeutic nurturance and support without fear of injury. Just as the chronically abused child may learn to avoid close interactions with potentially dangerous adults, the abuse survivor may use similar defenses that, at least initially, preclude a working relationship with his or her therapist. As many clinicians will attest, there is no shortcut to the process of developing trust in such instances. Instead, the clinician must provide ongoing reliable data to the survivor that he or she is not in danger—not from physical or sexual assaults, nor from rejection, domination, intrusion, or abandonment (Courtois, 1988; Meiselman, 1990; Salter, 1995).

Some therapists will agree to these principles but nevertheless unconsciously violate them. For instance, a clinician may spend considerable time reassuring the client that he or she is a safe and supportive person, yet at other times implicitly criticize, pathologize, or intrude on the survivor (Salter, 1995). Examples of such behavior are frequent interruptions, excessive clinical interpretations, ill-conceived confrontations, uninvited probing, and various forms of boundary violations. Alternatively, the therapist may violate the principles of good therapeutic process outlined earlier (e.g., pacing and intensity control), thereby communicating to the client that therapy is not, in fact, a safe place nor a process under the client's control. Such therapists may seek clinical consultation with complaints of client resistance or untreatable pathology, not realizing that his or her behavior in therapy may be motivating (or at least not lessening the need for) the client's responses.

In my experience, the therapist goes on record from the moment of the intake interview to the last treatment session. Has her behavior shown that vulnerability is possible without injury, criticism, or rejection? Does the client have any evidence that the clinician is prone to potentially abusive, neglectful, or boundary-violating behavior? Is it, ultimately, safe in the therapy office? These questions, constantly evaluated, form the base from which the abuse survivor will (or will not) respond to treatment interventions. When the answers consistently support the notion of safety, the survivor is more likely to "open up," and attempt new behaviors and experiences (Meiselman, 1990, 1994).

Beyond providing a secure base from which the client can explore his or her internal and interpersonal environment, therapeutic safety and support ideally provides a curative example of a relationship. Long-term interactions in a safe therapeutic relationship can rework previous assumptions about the value of self in relation to others, such that the client begins to approximate a sense of personal validity. By receiving continuous support from the therapist, the client has the opportunity to alter assumptions regarding what he or she is and could be, as well as to internalize the possibility of benevolent others and of situations for whom avoidance and defense are less required.

Facilitating Self-Awareness and Positive Identity

In the context of sustained and reliable support and acceptance, the survivor has the opportunity to engage in the relative luxury of introspection. Looking inward may have been punished by the survivor's early environment in at least two ways: It took attention away from hypervigilance and, therefore, safety, and greater internal awareness meant, by definition, greater pain. As a result, many untreated survivors of severe abuse are surprisingly unaware of their internal processes and logic, and may, in fact, appear to have little self-knowledge. This may present, for example, as reports of the inability to predict one's own behavior in various situations, or of little insight regarding the abuse or its effects. Some survivors refer to this knowledge gap as evidence of being "dumb" or "stupid": It is, of course, not a matter of intelligence, but rather of motivated avoidance and the psychological costs of survival-based other-directedness.

By facilitating self-exploration, abuse-focused therapy may allow the survivor to become more acquainted with self, and thus to gain a greater sense of personal identity. Increased self-awareness may be especially fostered by "Socratic therapy," wherein the client is asked many open-ended questions throughout the course of treatment. These include gentle questions about, for example, the client's early (preabuse) perceptions and experiences, the options that were and were not available to her at the time of the abuse, her current thoughts, feelings, and self-assessments, and her ongoing reactions to treatment. As opposed to the overuse of therapeutic interpretations or blanket reassurance, Socratic interventions not only support the survivor's acquisition of a growing body of information regarding the self, but also—and more important—teach the techniques of self-exploration and- examination. Thus, instead of learning about himself solely from the (implicitly wiser) therapist, the survivor develops the skills necessary to engage in the process of self-understanding on his own.

Self-Other and Boundary Issues

As noted earlier, many survivors of severe childhood sexual abuse have difficulty distinguishing the boundary between self and others. This problem is thought to arise both from attachment disruption, wherein the child is deprived of the opportunity to learn normal self-other behaviors, and from early intrusion by the abuser into the child's bodily space (McCann & Pearlman (1990).

Effective abuse-focused therapy addresses both of these bases. The clinician is careful to honor the client's dignity, rights, and psychological integrity—even if the survivor is unaware of his or her entitlement to such treatment. Over time, the therapist's consistent regard for the client's rights to safety and freedom from intrusion can be internalized by the client as evidence of her physical and psychological boundaries. Some of this learning process is cognitive—during the client's recounting of his child abuse history and later adult experiences of violation or exploitation, the therapist actively reinforces the survivor's previous and current entitlement to bodily and psychological integrity. Other aspects of this process are intrinsic—as she is treated with respect by the therapist, and slowly develops a growing sense of personal identity, the survivor begins to *assume* that she has outside limits and that these boundaries should not be violated by others.

At the same time that the demarcation of his or her own boundaries are being demonstrated and learned, the survivor in therapy may be exposed to important lessons regarding the boundaries of others. This may occur as the client impinges on the therapist, typically through inappropriate questions, requests, or expectations. As the therapist gently but firmly (and, it is hoped, adroitly) repels such intrusions, he or she both teaches about the needs and rights of others to boundary integrity, and models for the survivor appropriate limit-setting strategies the survivor can use in his or her own life. In this way, the interpersonal give-and-take of psychotherapy tends to replicate some of the lessons the survivor would have learned in childhood were it possible.

Affect Modulation and Affect Tolerance

Because affect tolerance and modulation are such important issues for adults severely abused as children, abuse-focused therapy addresses these issues in as many ways as possible. It stresses two general pathways to the development of affective competence: the acquisition of new affect regulation skills, and the strengthening of inborn, but underdeveloped, affective capacities.

Skills training in this area is well outlined by Linehan (1993) in her outstanding manual on the cognitive behavioral treatment of those with a diagnosis of borderline personality disorder. She notes that distress tolerance and emotional regulation are both internal behaviors that can, to some extent, be taught during therapy. Among the specific skills directly taught by Linehan's "dialectical behavior therapy" (DBT) for distress tolerance are distraction, self-soothing, "improving the moment" (e.g., through relaxation), and thinking of the "pros and cons" of behavior (p. 148). In the area of emotion regulation skills, Linehan teaches the survivor to, among other things, identify and label affect, identify obstacles to changing emotions, reduce vulnerability to hyperemotionality through decreased stress, increase the frequency of positive emotional events, and develop the ability to experience emotions without judging or rejecting them (pp. 147–148).

Abuse-focused therapy makes use of these skills training approaches, although it generally avoids the formally programmatic aspects of DBT. Linehan's (1993) model, which has been shown to be effective in outcome research (Linehan, 1993), stresses a central issue: affect regulation problems do not reflect a structural psychological defect (as suggested by some analytic theories and approaches) as much as insufficiently developed self-skills arising from distorted or disrupted childhood development.

Although somewhat less focused on concrete skill development than DBT, abuse-relevant therapy similarly focuses on the learning of affect regulation skills. First, as the survivor enters intense emotional states, the therapist regularly works with her to identify and describe her internal experience. This is an important step for some more severely abused individuals, who may be relatively unable to discriminate different feelings (e.g., anger from sadness from fear), and for whom the unknown and unpredictable qualities of intense affect produce feelings of chaos, helplessness, and further distress. Such individuals may respond to questions about internal experience by merely describing feeling "bad," without the apparent capacity to identify the relevant affect further. As the client becomes better able to label and describe feelings as they come up in treatment, he or she may become more "at home" with strong affect and less likely to fear emotionality as an unknown, unpredictable force.

Successful abuse-focused therapy also teaches the client how to maintain self-coherence and identity during strong affective states. As the client enters an especially powerful feeling state while, for example, describing a traumatic incident, the therapist may help him learn to "ground" himself: to focus attention on his biological functions (e.g., breathing and heart rate), physical sensations (e.g., the awareness of his feet on the floor or his body's contact with the chair), and external environment (e.g., the therapist's relaxed demeanor or the sound of nearby traffic). These grounding activities probably serve at least two functions: (a) they keep the survivor focused on her continued physical presence, such that she does not feel so caught up in emotional turmoil that she loses track of herself, and (b) they teach the survivor how to distract herself partially from overwhelming internal stimulation, thereby breaking the vicious cycle of escalating affect producing panic and further escalation.

The survivor also learns to identify and describe the intrusive and repetitive cognitions that often trigger and feed overwhelming affect. Thus, for example, the client's attention may be focused on the things she says to herself just before an emotional reactions (e.g., "he hates me," "they're trying to hurt me," or "I'm so disgusting"), and the cognitions occurring during the process of strong emotion that produce panic and fears of being overwhelmed or inundated (e.g., "I'm losing it," "I'm out of control," or "I'm making a fool of myself"). As the client becomes more aware of these cognitive antecedents to overwhelming affect, he or she can also learn to forestall such thoughts through "thought stopping," by disagreeing with herself (e.g., "nobody's out to get me," "I look/sound fine," or "I'm still in control; I can handle this"), or merely by experiencing such cognitions as old tapes rather than accurate perceptions.

Affect regulation and tolerance is also learned implicitly during abuse-focused therapy. Because, as outlined subsequently, trauma-focused interventions involve the repeated evocation and resolution of distressing but nonoverwhelming affect, such treatment slowly teaches the survivor to become more familiar with some level of nondissociated distress and to develop whatever skills are necessary to downwardly modulate emotional arousal. This growing ability to move in and out of strong affective states, in turn, fosters an increased sense of emotional control and reduced fear of affect. The reader is referred to McCann and Pearlman (1990, pp. 144–153) for further information on the development and strengthening of affect regulation capacities.

Intervening in Abuse-Related Trauma Symptoms

Assuming that the client either has sufficient self-skills or that these self-functions have been strengthened sufficiently, the treatment of trauma symptoms is relatively straightforward. There are at least three major steps in this process, although they may recur in different orders at various points in treatment: identification of traumatic (i.e., abuse-related) events; gradual reexposure to the affect and stimuli associated with a memory of the abuse, while keeping avoidance responses minimal; and emotional discharge and cognitive processing.

Identification of Traumatic Events

For traumatic material to be processed in treatment, it must be identified as such. Although this seems an obvious step, it is more difficult to implement in some cases than might be expected. As noted previously, the survivor's avoidance of abuse-related material may lead either to conscious reluctance to think about or speak of upsetting abuse incidents, or to less conscious dissociation of such events. In the former case, the survivor may believe that a detailed description of the abuse would be more painful than he or she is willing to endure, or that exploration of the abuse would overwhelm his or her self-resources. Dissociation of abuse material, conversely, may present as incomplete or absent recall of the events in question.

Whether denial or dissociation, avoidance of abuse-related material by the survivor should be respected because it indicates his or her judgment that exploration in that area would exceed the therapeutic window. The role of the therapist at such junctures is not to overpower the client's defenses or in any way to convince him or her that abuse occurred, but rather to provide the conditions (e.g., safety, support, and a trustworthy environment) whereby avoidance is less necessary. Because this latter step can require significant time and skill, the specific enumeration and description of abusive events is far from a simple matter (Courtois, 1995).

Gradual Exposure to Abuse-Related Material

If, at some point, there is sufficient abuse material available to the treatment process, the next step in the treatment of abuse-related trauma is that of careful, gradual exposure to various aspects of the abuse memory. According to Abueg and Fairbank (1992), exposure treatment can be defined as "repeated or extended exposure, either in vivo or in imagination, to objectively harmless but feared stimuli for the purpose of reducing anxiety" (p. 127). As noted earlier, the goal of exposure techniques in the current context is somewhat more ambitious than the mere eradication of irrational anxiety. Instead, the intended outcome includes the reduction of intrusive (and, secondarily, avoidant) symptomatology associated with unresolved traumatic events.

The exposure approach suggested here for abuse trauma is a form of systematic desensitization (Wolpe, 1958), wherein the survivor is asked to recall nonoverwhelming, but painful abuse-specific experiences in the context of a safe therapeutic environment and the positive effects of emotional discharge. The exposure is sequenced according to the intensity of the recalled abuse, with less upsetting memories being recalled and addressed in therapy before more upsetting ones are considered. The use of exposure or desensitization procedures appears to be effective in the treatment of various types of trauma survivors, including rape victims (Foa, Rothbaum, Riggs, & Murdock, 1991; Frank & Stewart, 1983) and war veterans (Bowen & Lambert, 1986; Keane, Fairbank, Caddell, & Zimering, 1989).

In contrast to more strictly behavioral interventions, however, abused-focused psychotherapy does not adhere to a strict, pre-planned series of exposure activities. This is due, in part, to the fact that most survivors in therapy present with a complex history of multiple and chronic abusive and neglectful acts that occurred many years ago as opposed to a single instance of rape or other assault during adulthood. Further, the survivor's ability to tolerate exposure may vary considerably from session to session as a function of his or her level of self-capacities, extent of outside life stressors, level of support from friends, relatives, and others, and the "place" in the therapeutic window that the therapy occupies at any given moment. In addition, the immediate target for desensitization may not be a discrete memory, but rather the more elusive and complex phenomenon of transferentially evoked abuse-relevant thoughts and feelings. In fact, as noted in chapter 4, transference is a frequent and powerful form of abuse reexperiencing, and thus is a potent source of nonspecific but important material that can be desensitized during treatment.

Regarding the last point, the client may be sufficiently stressed by previous therapeutic events or transferential aspects of the therapeutic relationship (e.g., the restimulated attachment dynamics described in chapter 5) that his or her ability to handle any further stressful material is limited. Further processing of abuse memories or responses at such times usually leads to avoidance, or even to some level of fragmentation. As a result, the focus of therapy becomes consolidation, arousal reduction (e.g., via grounding), and the shoring up of self-resources as indicated in the earlier "process" section of this chapter. In addition, if exploration of abuse-related issues has led to enduring feelings of revulsion, self-hatred, or helplessness, the client may require interventions that interrupt or contradict cognitive distortions before he or she can move on to more exposure.

As noted by McCann and Pearlman (1990), exposure to abuse memories is complicated by the fact that there are probably at least two different memory systems to address: verbal and imagery (although we later refer to the latter as "sensorimotor"). The former is more narrative and autobiographical, whereas the latter involves the encoding and recovery of sensations and nonverbal experiences. McCann and Pearlman (1990) note that material from both systems must be desensitized—the first by repeatedly exploring the factual aspects of the event (e.g., who, what, where, and when), and the second by recollection and recounting of the physical environment and bodily sensations associated with the abuse. In my experience, processing of verbal memories is considerably less overwhelming for most survivors than exploration of sensory memories; therefore, the former should usually be addressed around any given memory before the latter is elicited.

The need to process sensory material may be especially relevant because, as indicated by van der Kolk (1994) and others, it is likely that some components of posttraumatic memory are intrinsically sensory or sensorimotor. As a result, therapeutic work that focuses solely on the narrative level (i.e., as is seen in some intellectualized therapies) is unlikely to allow processing of all available posttraumatic material. In contradistinction, good trauma work is both cognitive and affective—addressing not only distorted cognitions and the acquisition of insight, but also the need for emotional expression, processing, and desensitization.

As indicated earlier, for abuse-focused therapy to work well, there should be as little avoidance as possible during the session. Specifically, the client should be encouraged to stay as "present" as he or she can during the detailed recall of abuse memories, so that desensitization is maximized. The extremely dissociated survivor may have little true exposure to abuse material during treatment—despite what may be detailed verbal renditions of a given memory. The therapist must keep the therapeutic window in mind, and not, however, interrupt survivor dissociation that is, in fact, appropriate in the face of therapeutic overstimulation. This might occur, for example, when the client accesses memories whose affective characteristics exceed his or her self-resources. Conversely, it is not uncommon for dissociative responses to become so overlearned that they automatically (but unnecessarily) emerge during exploration of stressful material. In this case, some level of encouragement of the client to reduce his or her dissociation during treatment is not only safe but frequently imperative for significant desensitization to occur.

Emotional Processing

The last component of abuse-focused desensitization of trauma involves the emotional activity that must occur during self-exposure to traumatic memories. This is an important step because, without such processing, exposure may result only in reexperienced pain, not resolution of symptoms (Rachman, 1980). In other words, therapeutic interventions that focus solely on the reporting of abuse-related memories will not necessarily produce symptom relief. There are two aspects of emotional processing immediately relevant to the treatment of severe abuse trauma: facilitation of emotional discharge and titration of level of affect.

Effective abuse-related therapy capitalizes on the positive effects of emotional release. In this regard, crying and other forms of emotional discharge may operate as inborn healing/countercondition-ing responses. Specifically, emotional release (e.g., crying, raging, and screaming) may countercondition (neutralize) the pain initially associated with the trauma by pairing the memory with emotional relief, thereby inhibiting its linkage with distress. In other words, the common suggestion that someone "have a good cry" or "get it off of your chest" may reflect folk-wisdom support for ventilation and other emotional activities that naturally desensitize trauma. From this perspective, just as traditional systematic desensitization pairs a formerly distressing stimulus to a relaxed (anxiety-incom-patible) state, and thereby neutralizes the original anxious response over time, repeated emotional discharge during nondissociated exposure to painful memories allows the processing of traumatic stimuli in the context of the relatively positive internal states asso-ciated with emotional release. Thus, a "good cry" is good because, in the absence of significant dissociation, it tends to allow counter-conditioning of traumatic material.

Although appropriate emotional expression may facilitate the desensitization of abuse-related trauma, such activity is not equivalent to the recently rediscovered notion of "abreaction" of chronic abuse trauma. These more dramatic procedures often involve pressure on the client to engage in extreme emotional discharge, sometimes in response to previously unavailable material, often in the context of an hypnotic state. Unfortunately, such techniques run the risk of greatly exceeding the therapeutic window, with resultant flooding of painful affects. In addition, by their very nature, such interventions encourage dissociated emotional release—a phenomenon that, although easily accomplished by many survivors, is unlikely to be therapeutically helpful. As noted by Cornell and Olio (1991), "[abreactive] techniques may appear to deepen affect and produce dramatic results in the session, but they may not result in the client's sustained understanding of, or connection to, their experience of abuse" (p. 62).

The nondissociated emotional processing of abuse-related traumatic response can, therefore, be seen as a natural—albeit sometimes painful—way to metabolize posttraumatic stress psychologically. The survivor who remembers her abuse (both narratively and through intrusive sensory reexperiencing), who cries or rages about it, and who repetitively talks and ruminates about it is engaging in a natural healing response. For many survivors, this process may best occur during therapy, where the clinician can provide a safe and organized structure for the unfolding of each component and can be counted on to keep the processing well within the therapeutic window. As noted earlier, the survivor's existing self-resources will determine how much exposure and processing can occur without overwhelming her and stimulating avoidance responses.

Access to Previously Unavailable Material

Taken together, the approach outlined thus far allows the therapist to address the impaired self-functioning and posttraumatic stress found in some adults who were severely abused as children. The slow desensitization of painful memories is likely to reduce the survivor's overall level of posttraumatic stress—a condition that eventually lessens the overall level of avoidance required by the survivor for internal stability. This process also increases self-resources—as noted earlier, progressive exposure to nonoverwhelming distress is likely to increase the development of affect regulation skills and affect tolerance. As a result, successful ongoing treatment allows the survivor to confront increasingly more painful memories without exceeding the survivor's (now greater) self-capacities.

In combination, decreasing stress levels and increasing self-resources can lead to a relatively self-sustaining process: As the need to avoid painful material lessens, memories previously too overwhelming to address become more available for processing. As this new material is, in turn, desensitized and cognitively accommodated, self-capacity is further improved, and the overall stress level is further reduced—thereby permitting access to (and processing of) even more unavailable material. Ultimately, treatment ends when traumatic material is sufficiently desensitized and integrated, and self-resources are sufficiently learned and strengthened, so that the survivor no longer experiences significant abuse-related intrusive, avoidant, or dysphoric symptoms.

This progressive function of abuse-focused therapy removes the need for any so-called memory recovery techniques. Instead of relying on hypnosis or drug-assisted interviews, for example, to somehow increase access to unavailable ("unconscious" or "repressed") material, this approach allows these memories to emerge naturally as a function of the survivor's reduced need for avoidance. Authoritarian memory recovery techniques might easily exceed the therapeutic window and flood the survivor with destabilizing and potentially injurious memories and affects, whereas appropriate abuse-focused therapy only allows access to dissociated material when, by definition, the therapeutic window has not been exceeded. The treatment model presented here reverses an assumption of those who advocate aggressive memory retrieval: It holds that clients do not get better when they remember more but rather that they may remember more as they get better.

Intervening in Distorted Cognitions

In the process of self-exploration and the desensitization of trauma-related affects and recollections, many opportunities arise for the reworking of cognitive distortions and negative self-perceptions. Beyond the cognitive processes that underlie overwhelming emotionality, described earlier, these distortions typically involve harsh self-judgments of having caused, encouraged, or deserved the abuse (Jehu, Gazan, & Klassen, 1984–85), as well as those broader self-esteem problems typically associated with child maltreatment (Briere, 1992). In many cases, in fact, it appears that complete emotional processing requires cognitive processing of abuse-related thoughts as well. Resick and Schnicke (1993), for example, note that "Prolonged exposure [i.e., recollection of the abuse] activates the memory structure but does not provide corrective information regarding misattributions or other maladaptive beliefs" (p. 17). By exploring with the survivor the inadequate information and logical errors associated with such beliefs and self-perceptions, the therapist can assist in the development of a more positive model of self and more complete resolution of traumatic stress.

Many victims of socially prevalent abuse paradoxically feel ashamed, believing that they or their experiences were abnormal (Coates & Winston, 1983). Typical of this stigmatization dynamic (Finkelhor & Browne, 1985) are survivor statements, such as: "There must be something wrong with me to have had this happen," or "I feel different from everyone else—I can't tell them what happened." This sense of shame and isolation can be especially profound for the sexual abuse survivor because, in many cases, he was directly told as a child that he was to blame, that the abuse reflected something about him, and that he must keep his victimization a secret.

In response to the survivor's experience of abnormality, many therapeutic approaches to abuse trauma focus on *normalization* as a primary technique. Normalization refers to therapist interventions that help the survivor to understand that her current behavior is not irrational or abnormal but rather an entirely understandable reaction to her childhood experience. One of the most direct forms of normalization occurs when the therapist shares information with the client regarding (a) the relative commonness of abuse in our society, and thus the fact that he or she is not alone; (b) the abuser's and society's (not the victim's) culpability regarding the molestation and its impact; and (c) the common psychological effects of sexual abuse.

The last, although risking the possibility of pathologizing the survivor or prescribing symptoms if not done well, often provides her with the first inkling of the fact that abuse (not her inherent weakness or badness) has logical and predictable effects. Such information should not be presented as if the survivor will necessarily experience every problem described but rather should convey the notion that her difficulties represent known (and therefore not idiosyncratic) psychological phenomena. Especially useful in this regard is early discussion of the symptoms of PTSD as they relate to sexual victimization and the more specific aspects of post–sexual-abuse trauma as described in this book and elsewhere. Again, the intent of this exercise is to explain current or future problems, not to prescribe them.

In addition to providing information, the clinician may need to engage in more formal cognitive therapy regarding the client's feelings of abnormality, shame, and isolation elicited by reexperienced abuse phenomena. Among other things, this may involve asking the client to describe concretely those thoughts or interpretations of memories that cause him to feel as if he is intrinsically bad or different from others. When these cognitions are described, for example, "What we did was horrible, and I know that people would be disgusted with me if they found out," the therapist may gently work with the survivor to disentangle the connection between bad things happening to her and her being bad.

This process does not, however, involve the therapist lecturing the client on her "illogical thinking" as much as it reflects a spirit of "why is it that when A happens to us, we often think B, and end up feeling/doing C?" The intent of such clarification is the client's growing awareness of the negative assumptions she makes regarding the meaning of the abuse, both in terms of how she sees herself and how she construes her value to others. In this way, the therapist may respectfully and gently challenge the client's abuse-related assumptions and provide the necessary questions and feedback to permit her to reexamine these beliefs. As is true of cognitive therapy for other problems, such interventions must be accompanied by consistent support and patience because abuse-related beliefs are often slow to change. The eventual result, however, especially in a therapeutic environment that avoids criticism or blame, is well worth the effort.

SOME FINAL COMMENTS ON ABUSE-RELATED PSYCHOTHERAPY

This chapter has integrated those aspects of current dynamic, cognitive, and behavioral approaches that may be helpful in the treatment of severe abuse trauma. It suggests that postabuse symptomatology generally reflects the survivor's adaptive attempts to maintain internal stability in the face of potentially overwhelming abuse-related pain. It further suggests that many of these symptoms are, in actuality, inborn self-healing procedures that only fail when overwhelming stress or inadequate internal resources motivate the overuse of avoidance activities.

Successful treatment for abuse-related distress and dysfunction should not seek to impose alien techniques and perspectives on the survivor, but rather should help the client to do better what he or she is already attempting to do. Thus, like the survivor, the therapist should be especially concerned with balancing challenge with resource and growth with safety. The natural healing aspects of intrusion and avoidance are not countered in treatment, but instead are refined to the point that they are maximally helpful and can be abandoned once successful.

As was noted at the beginning of this chapter, and despite the various methods and techniques presented previously, probably the most important components of psychotherapy with abuse survivors involve its most generic aspects: a therapist who is caring, nonexploitive, and reliable, and a safe therapeutic environment that fosters self-awareness, self-acceptance, and the careful processing of traumatic material. Thus, the corrective interpersonal experience of abuse-focused psychotherapy is as much about how the therapist is as it is what he or she says.

The Specific Problem of Client Dissociation During Therapy

7

In some ways, psychotherapy represents a paradox for the sexual abuse survivor: On the one hand, she has been victimized and exploited in the context of an interpersonal relationship. On the other, it is suggested that her best chance for recovery may be to engage in a similar situation where, she is told, she should "trust" that further abuse will not occur.

From the survivor's perspective, there are several communalities between her abuse and psychotherapy: Both involve a form of intimate relationship with an authority figure, both can be emotionally painful, and both demand vulnerability. These similarities, in combination with the survivor's almost reflexive hypervigilance and general distrust, make it difficult for some former abuse victims to (a) attend psychotherapy and (b) stay there. It is with regard to the latter point that this chapter is written: Just as during her abuse the victim used dissociative strategies to leave the scene of her trauma psychologically, so may the adult survivor dissociate from the psychotherapeutic process at times of stress or perceived danger.

Such dissociative behaviors can be unconscious defensive strategies and yet autonomous "symptoms," and can emerge in either primitive or more sophisticated forms. Some dissociative states may be obvious to the client, the therapist, or both, whereas others may be considerably more subtle and may not be recognizable as dissociative by either member of the psychotherapy dyad.

Whatever its form, as described in chapter 6, extreme or chronic dissociation can significantly reduce the effectiveness of psychotherapy. Among other possible effects, dissociation during therapy may

- *Reduce the survivor's exposure to recollected abusive events,* thereby decreasing the opportunity to process them in treatment. If the survivor keeps from fully recalling an aversive event, for example, he may not have a chance to associate this memory with current positive therapeutic experiences (e.g., emotional discharge, or the experience of current safety and support) that facilitate its desensitization and will not be able to alter those distorted cognitive responses associated with the abuse.
- *Reduce the amount of anxiety and distress felt during the session,* so that it cannot fade away (habituate) in the absence of reinforcement. In the absence of avoidance, the repeated elicitation of a conditioned emotional response without the expected outcome (e.g., feeling fear without there being any danger) often causes that emotional response to decrease over time. From this perspective, the survivor who numbs herself while recalling a childhood assault may miss the opportunity to habituate the associated anxiety in the safety of the therapy environment.
- *Reinforce continued avoidance responses.* Because dissociation is usually effective to some extent in reducing the experience of psychic pain, its use is continually reinforced. Thus, the survivor who avoids recollecting or feeling abuse-related trauma is rewarded with decreased distress. This negative reinforcement can be powerful and may easily generalize to other stressful situations. As a result, the survivor may dissociate more frequently and more automatically, including during treatment.
- *Cause the survivor to miss important therapeutic events,* such as the opportunity to develop insight or to become emotionally connected with the therapist. A client who is functionally "not there" during therapy will miss many of its benefits.
- *Preclude the development of greater affect regulation skills.* The use of dissociation during treatment reduces the possibility of developing greater affect tolerance because the client generally avoids the full experience of negative affect and, therefore, is not challenged to develop greater emotional resilience. Similarly, the survivor is less

likely to learn new ways to modulate painful affect given the power of dissociation to regulate distress downwardly.

Although each of the preceding points represent ways in which dissociation can hinder recovery, the survivor may have little choice but to do so. Dissociative response can represent a vicious cycle wherein abuse-related psychic pain is reduced through dissociation, yet the continued use of dissociation precludes the development of other ways of dealing with or resolving psychic pain. In this way, dissociation begets dissociation. As a result, it is rarely a simple matter of somehow causing the abuse survivor to dissociate less during a specific session. In fact, heavy-handed therapist attempts to reduce client dissociation may easily exceed the therapeutic window, thereby overwhelming the client and motivating further dissociation.

Given the frequency of dissociation in abuse-related psychotherapy, its resistance to direct intervention, and its impact on the treatment process, this phenomenon is addressed in detail in the following pages. First, six common forms of therapy-based dissociation are presented and their typical impacts on treatment are noted, and then a general approach to dealing with therapy-based dissociation is discussed.

COMMON FORMS OF THERAPY-BASED DISSOCIATION

Disengagement

Disengagement is probably the simplest and most common form of dissociation. Invoked by most people on occasion, this defense—sometimes referred to as "spacing out"—involves a cognitive separation of the individual from his or her environment at times of stress. This disengagement from the external world is not to be confused with daydreaming or distraction by other thoughts or affects. Instead, the individual withdraws into a state of cognitive neutrality, where thoughts are seemingly "placed on hold." During such times, he or she may be temporarily unresponsive to conversation or questions, although he will usually "snap out of it" if the questioner persists in seeking his attention. Most periods of cognitive disengagement are relatively brief, ranging from a few seconds to usually less than several minutes, and the depth of the dissociation is typically shallow.

As opposed to most nonvictimized persons, the survivor of severe abuse may slip in and out of disengagement many times a day, apparently in an attempt to titrate the stress of daily living down to manageable levels. These frequent and brief "time-outs" are often not recognized as such by the individual, who may be surprised to hear from others that he or she is inattentive during discussions or other interpersonal interactions.

The defensive aspects of cognitive disengagement reside in the survivor's ability to attenuate psychologically disturbing or threatening stimuli—whether they be internally generated (e.g., flashbacks, painful memories, or intrusive thoughts) or encountered in the interpersonal environment (e.g., real or perceived danger, and boundary violations). Like many other psychological defenses, disengagement usually occurs as a function of unconscious decision making: The individual perceives a potential threat that exceeds or stresses internal self-resources, and "decides" to cognitively withdraw as a protection against sustained anxiety and other painful affects commonly associated with trauma. Because disengagement is rarely planned at the conscious level, and its net effect is to decrease awareness, the survivor may not notice that she is dissociating until after the fact—if at all.

The primary impact of disengagement in therapy is that the client may miss important insights or opportunities for self-awareness while "away." Such interference is especially likely in the early stages of abuse-oriented treatment, when the survivor is most fearful of the therapist and therapy, although it may reemerge as a problem at later times of stress.

Detachment/Numbing

As opposed to disengagement, detachment does not require the survivor to avoid current experiencing cognitively; instead, he or she figuratively "turns down the volume control" of negative feelings associated with certain thoughts, memories, or events, so that the latter may be engaged in with less emotional pain. This defense, like disengagement, is used by most people at one time or another as a way of handling acute stress, grief, anger, or other aversive states. Typically in the survivor, however, detachment (also referred to as "numbing") serves as a primitive protection from the painful sequelae of child abuse or as a regular defense against affective responses to current abuse-related events (e.g., the numbness frequently associated with prostitution or chronic physical abuse in marriage).

Although often adaptive in dealing with acute or immediate traumatic experiences, recurrent or sustained forms of detachment (as is found, for example, in chronic PTSD and some dissociative disorders) can easily interfere with the psychic processing of painful affect. In its chronic incarnation, this numbing may result in an individual who is psychologically removed from her feelings and who may, in fact, be relatively unaware of feelings. Such people, especially if they have had access to a university education, may present in an intellectualized manner, using verbal and analytic skills to turn subjective (personal) distress into "objective" (impersonal) data. Typical statements of clients whose use of detachment is automatic and largely unconscious may include "I feel dead inside," "I don't feel bad about what he did—I understand that, on some level, he must have been a very disturbed and alienated person," or "I know in my mind that I must be upset, but I can't feel it."

The primary effect of detachment on psychotherapy is that the client may fail to resolve traumatic material. By keeping painful feelings out of consciousness during affective processing of abuse issues, the survivor is unable to countercondition or habituate them. The net result may be someone with exceptionally good insight into the various aspects of her victimization, perhaps even into her own reactions and accommodations to the abuse, who nevertheless continues to feel suppressed and unacknowledged rage, sadness, and fear regarding these events and her role in them.

Dissociative Observation

This phenomenon is often described by clients as watching oneself engage in an interaction, as opposed actually to participating in

it. In this sense, observation has much in common with the depersonalization and out-of-body experiences found in abuse survivors
and other PTSD sufferers. The primary difference between the current defense and these other dissociative states is that the latter
occur as relatively sudden, discrete episodes, whereas observation
is a chronic pattern of avoiding the direct experience of stressful
events. The client will frequently describe a feeling of calm or affective neutrality, which can be traced to a sense of being "outside looking in" and, therefore, not directly threatened by whatever potentially frightening stimulus is present. Thus, observation may also be
understood as another pathway to detachment, where separation
from affect is accomplished by, at least metaphorically, distancing
oneself from the stressor.

In the therapy session, observation serves to divorce affect from
thought in much the same way as does detachment. As an observer
of psychotherapy, rather than as a participant, the client can be relatively uninvolved in the treatment process and thus less "touched"
by it. The problem with this solution to therapy-based emotional
pain is that by removing one's self from treatment, one cannot benefit much from the process. Dissociated distress is much more difficult to habituate, desensitize, or otherwise process. Luckily for most
survivors, the observer defense is less frequently used as treatment
progresses, especially if, as described later, the clinician actively
addresses this problem during therapy

Intersession Discontinuity

A frequent experience of therapists working with survivors of
severe abuse is that their clients seem to approach some sessions as
if they had never been in earlier ones. The client may, for example,
not recall important material uncovered in the previous therapy
meeting, may deny that the clinician ever said certain things, or may
cover "new" ground that was identically addressed in one or more
earlier sessions. In the last edition of this book, this phenomenon
was referred to as "postsession amnesia." It is relabeled in this edition because the phenomenon is broader than only memory gaps
between sessions—most generally it reflects a defensive separation
or discontinuity between sessions.

This behavior can be understood in several different ways: (a) It could be that the client is unable to maintain "object constancy" from session to session, and thus she is, in fact, beginning anew in each session; (b) it could be that the client was inattentive in previous sessions, as a result of various dissociative defenses, and thus did not "receive" information that was available at a given point in time; or (c) it is possible that the client has, for whatever reason, forgotten or cognitively avoided what transpired in certain therapeutic interactions.

Although all three of these dynamics may operate in the abuse survivor, the third notion—that of avoiding recent therapy material—often underlies what appears to be session-to-session discontinuity. Specifically, just as psychogenic amnesia is understood to be a dissociative phenomenon in current diagnostic systems (i.e., DSM-IV), so too may the client use dissociative techniques to eliminate what otherwise might be growing awareness of threatening material during the treatment process.

Thus, for example, the client might not recall an insight developed in the previous session that her father did not, in fact, truly love her or may avoid newly accessed memories of having taken money or candies for "not telling" about an abuse episode. In the former instance, discontinuity protects the survivor from confronting the full extent of her exploitation and betrayal, whereas in the latter case it may forestall guilt arising from the belief that she gained from her molestation.

Finally, intrasession discontinuity can serve to break up the flow of the therapeutic process for the survivor, allowing him to (a) titrate the intensity and rate of treatment and (b) moderate the extent of closeness or dependency on his therapist. In this regard, the discontinuity of therapy that may arise is, in fact, the unconsciously planned outcome.

As If

This defense is perhaps the most sophisticated form of dissociation found among sexual abuse survivors. Deployment of "as if" dissociation in therapy can result in a client who appears to be present during treatment, who engages in spontaneous, "real"-appearing affect (e.g., tears or anger), but who never seems to improve or gain emotional insight into his or her experience. Careful examination of such individuals, however, may reveal that their participation is "too good to be true," and that there is a subtle sense of unconscious play acting about their presentation. It may appear, for example, that the survivor is an excellent performer of a script that requires one to act as if she were a client, with all the attendant emotions and behaviors that role requires.

The relative sophistication of this defense lies in its subtlety: "as if" may interfere with the treatment process without either the clinician or the client being aware of it. The underlying unconscious strategy appears to be the following: "I cannot allow myself to experience the pain and fear that go along with confronting and fully feeling my distress, and the process of psychotherapy itself is frightening (especially given my previous experience with the results of intimacy). However, I want to be good for this powerful other, and I want to believe that I am involved in a process that will help me. Therefore, I will play the part of myself being in therapy: I will get angry, cry, remember things, and report on them, but it won't be me—it will be me playing the part of me. The difference between these two states is enough to keep me safe and to keep me in control."

It has often been noted that therapy with those identified as having a borderline or histrionic personality disorder may superficially progress quite well early in treatment, yet later sessions may stall as it becomes clear that the client was not "really" working in therapy after all. Although such outcomes may derive from several different sources, one frequent factor appears to be the "as if" dissociative defense described here, especially when such clients are survivors of severe sexual abuse. In these instances, the client may be understood as attempting to survive psychotherapy psychologically—not trying to trick the therapist or undermine the treatment process, but rather, attempting to be present and not present, be a good client and yet still safe.

As is true of other dissociative defenses, the "as if" response interferes with the processing of traumatic memory and affect by reducing the survivor's actual contact with the evocative aspects of treatment. Because this defense is so subtle, at least in some instances, the "as if" client and her therapist may not easily understand why such reliably "good work" is not leading to any demonstrable therapeutic progress over time.

Dissociative Withdrawal

"As if" is a relatively complex form of dissociation, whereas dissociative withdrawal (referred to as "shutdown" in the last version of this book) is more primitive.

> Elaine is an obese, 31-year-old woman who has been in therapy for 6 months. As a child, she was a victim of extensive sadistic abuse, involving long periods of being tied to a bed, raped with various objects, and burned with cigarettes. Elaine appears to be doing well in treatment and is already gaining some control over the substance addiction and dissociative periods that have plagued her adult life.
>
> During her current session, however, Elaine becomes increasingly unresponsive and psychologically distant, apparently in response to an especially powerful series of flashbacks to her childhood torture. At one point her eyes roll up into her head, her eyelids flutter, and she begins to moan and cry. Her arms are rigidly folded across her chest, and she slides off her chair into a fetal position on the floor. Elaine is nonresponsive to her therapist's questions as she slowly rocks back and forth, and side to side. After about 15 minutes, she gradually "returns" to the room and sits back on her chair. She remains withdrawn, however, and it is not until her next session that she is able to discuss her experience, which she characterizes as a humiliating fall into a "black hole" of terror and seeming loss of volition.

Typically invoked when the client feels out of control or unable to avoid overwhelming affect, dissociative withdrawal involves movement into a mute, seemingly catatonic state during treatment. Although it shares many features with disengagement, dissociative withdrawal is not a retreat into neutrality; it appears to be an autistic wrestling with frightening cognitions or affects, motivating a need to stop most levels of awareness. As with other defensive strategies, this dissociative mechanism occurs on a continuum: ranging from short-term, diminished awareness of the clinician, self, and the psychotherapeutic environment to more extended periods of seemingly catatonic behavior, often (although not always) with attendant rocking and moaning or crying. The intent of such behaviors, over which the client often feels no conscious control, is sensory "shutdown" and escape from an overwhelmingly threatening internal environment. That a person would experience such elemental terror or pain during psychotherapy emphasizes the severity of her injury. That she would feel the need to engage in such primitive behaviors and yet not physically escape the therapy office underlines the extreme sense of helplessness and dependency the survivor may experience.

DYNAMIC TENSION BETWEEN DISSOCIATION AND PSYCHOTHERAPY

The major impediment of dissociation to effective psychotherapy is the fact that one acts in direct cross-purpose to the other. Primary goals of abuse-focused psychotherapy are exposure and integration: the simultaneous awareness and availability of thought and feelings, of "contradictory" or threatening states. Dissociation, conversely, is specific in its drive for avoidance and disintegration. Detachment serves to emphasize thought and deny affect, "as if" can involve the reverse, and disengagement separates the person from her outside world. Multiple personalities (dissociative identity disorder) and other forms of splitting go even further, disintegrating various parts of awareness so that all are separate but incomplete. The bottom line of each of these defenses is equivalent: By reducing or compartmentalizing access to threatening feelings or awareness, the survivor can continue to exist without being overwhelmed by abuse-related phenomena.

Psychotherapy, conversely, implies the contrary. It assumes that only reexperienced trauma can be processed, and that greater self-awareness often leads to self-acceptance. Thus, the therapy session may figuratively resemble a battleground: The therapist invites the client to experience and understand truly, whereas the client works—through various dissociative and avoidant defenses—to avoid what he believes to be dangerous affects and self-knowledge. Paraphrasing a 52-year-old actor, midpoint in therapy: "I don't trust you or me enough to open doors where I've locked in monsters. I'm supposed to believe you that this will help, but you can't help me if you're wrong."

Intervention

According to the general principles of treatment outlined in this book, the clinician is advised to view dissociation as a survival response to be respected rather than a symptom to be removed or discounted. Instead of being told merely to "stop dissociating" or "pay attention," the client is asked to (a) attend to her dissociative behavior (much of which may be out of her conscious awareness); and (b) if possible, reduce her dissociation to its most minimal, yet effective, level. If dissociation continues, it is assumed that the avoidance level is appropriate for the moment—that dissociation is serving to reduce traumatic stress to the point that it can be accommodated by existing self-capacities. In this instance, the therapist assumes that the therapeutic window is exceeded and works to (a) reduce the client's immediate level of stress or (b) increase her level of self-support.

Fortunately, it is often the case that the client's therapy-based dissociative behavior is, to some extent, reflexive and overlearned, and thus she may be able to reduce this impediment to treatment with only minor difficulty. For this reason, the two major therapeutic responses to dissociation emphasize awareness and control. For the purpose of discussion, these are referred to as *process feedback* and *self-monitoring*.

Process feedback refers to the therapist's continuing attention to the possibility of client dissociation (signaled by behaviors, such as fixed or "glazed" eyes, sudden flattening of affect, long lapses between words, monotone verbalizations, stereotyped gestures, seemingly "unreal" responses, or excessive intellectualization), and her gentle reminders to the client when such dissociation occurs. This feedback is not expressed punitively or in a negative way, but more in the manner of a team member informing her partner of an impending problem. Typical examples might be, "Jim, are you still with me? Are you going away?" or "Sarah, you seem to be spacing out a bit. Is something going on?" Inherent in the clinician's comments, regardless of their content, should be the message that dissociation is not an inherently bad response, only one that has a "downside" and should be monitored for its immediate appropriateness. In fact, punitive or castigating therapist reactions in this area often *increase* client dissociation, as the survivor struggles to distance herself further from abusive contact.

On being informed or reminded of dissociation by their therapists, most clients are able to at least temporarily reduce disengagement, detachment, or observation. If the client continues to have problems "returning" (especially in the case of disengagement or observation), the clinician may help the survivor ground herself by inviting her to pay attention to her bodily feelings, contact with the chair and ground, and describable stimuli in the immediate environment. Similarly, clients who become too detached may benefit from support for catharsis and "feeling your feelings." In many cases, such intervention may merely consist of frequently asking one's client "What are you feeling now?" "How does it feel when you say that?" or "It looks like there's a feeling in there somewhere. Do you know what it is?"

Less easily confronted, as might be expected, is the "as if" defense. In many cases this form of dissociation may go unnoticed by both therapist and client. Even when detected, however, "as if" may be difficult to derail because it is not always clear exactly what it is that the client is doing. Perhaps the most effective intervention is simply to educate the client about the "as if" phenomenon, point out to him instances in which it may be occurring (this should always be phrased tentatively because a process this subtle may be misidentified), and work with him to "make the session real" in any way that seems to work. Among the latter possibilities are (a) grounding techniques; (b) increased focus on feelings; and (c) gentle reminders that therapy is for the client, not the therapist, and can be paced accordingly. Given the ambiguity of this defense and the lack of clear solutions to its presence, it is reassuring to note that "as if," like other treatment-based dissociative events, tends to decrease as psychotherapy continues over time—especially if dissociation is directly, gently, and continually addressed during treatment.

Extreme dissociative withdrawal is undoubtedly the most frustrating and, in some cases, the most frightening of the dissociative responses. Not only is the client seemingly "not home" to receive therapeutic contact, the drama of a psychologically absent person may prove overwhelming to some clinicians. Common labels used for such client behavior include "catatonic" (in the schizophrenic sense), "regressed," "autistic," and "psychotic"—all descriptions that imply extremely negative prognoses. Thus, perhaps the first intervention the therapist may wish to consider is the decatastrophizing of his or her own cognitions. Dissociative withdrawal is an avoidance defense, not a psychotic break. Even when untreated, it is self-limiting—most instances of this phenomenon last for minutes; relatively few endure for more than several hours.

It is my experience that most clients are not totally "absent," even during extreme withdrawal. There is often a part of the client's awareness that remains focused on the environment for self-protective purposes and thus is somewhat accessible to the clinician. The therapist may find it helpful to talk to this part, even though the survivor appears nonresponsive. Typically, the therapist's statements at this time should be reassuring, normalizing, stress reducing, and nondemanding of response. The client may be told, for example: "We've gone far enough today; now we just need to get you back and together for the outside world, when you're ready," or "Sarah, it looks as if you've got a lot of stuff happening inside. I think we should just wait a while and let things settle down before we move on." Finally, the clinician should be alert to the possibility that what appears to be dissociative withdrawal is, instead, volitional nonresponse. The client may, in other words, be involved in instrumental activities to alter the therapist's behavior. He may, for example, be fearful of the material being discussed, or may be angry at the psychotherapist for real or imagined failings.

Extreme dissociative withdrawal is best discriminated from active nonresponse in terms of the client's awareness of her environment. Withdrawal may manifest with glazed, fixed, or closed eyes; rocking; rigid or tense musculature; and other signs of less voluntary activity. Volitional nonresponse may involve glaring, turning of the head away or downward, sudden nonverbal responses to further therapist statements, a grim or stubborn-appearing mien, and other evidence of ongoing awareness.

Because abuse-focused therapy actively involves the client in the recovery process, a final aspect of intervention relies on the client's self-monitoring of her or his dissociative processes. The survivor slowly learns to recognize times when he is reflexively distancing himself from frightening stimuli or affects. As he becomes more aware of the archaic quality of many of his fears and reactions, and as therapy works to reduce traumatic stress and increase self-capacities, such treatment-related dissociative episodes and processes become increasingly ego dystonic and lose much of their reinforcing quality. In turn, decreased dissociation increases the power of therapy to desensitize trauma and thus further reduce the need for dissociation.

In closing, it should be reiterated that dissociation during the therapy session may be entirely appropriate and should not necessarily be discouraged. Early in treatment, the survivor may need to reduce contact with painful internal experience as a way to keep from being overwhelmed by therapeutic restimulation of abuse-related trauma. Attempts to somehow force the survivor to give up avoidance prematurely almost inherently exceed the therapeutic window and potentially increase—rather than decrease—abuse-related distress and avoidance.

Teasing the Dragon: The Fruits of Confronting Severe Abuse

8

There are several ancient Eastern teaching tales with the same basic story: A person disturbs a slumbering beast, usually a tiger or a dragon. On awakening, the beast becomes angry and dangerous. The person thus finds herself faced with a conflict: to hang onto the beast (by the tail) means exposure to a frightening ride but potentially (at some point in the future) a positive outcome; to let go is to stop the ride but also to become vulnerable to an awakened and angry creature.

This chapter is about such a dilemma as it relates to work with more severely injured abuse survivors: "Awakening" the survivor's often dissociated or otherwise avoided awareness of extreme childhood trauma, as well as restimulating unresolved attachment dynamics, may cause her to feel and appear as if she is "getting worse" while in treatment. As psychotherapy supports the gradual exploration and reexperiencing of previously avoided awareness, memories, unmet childhood needs, and abuse-related affects, the survivor may experience a subjective increase in dysphoria. This increase in distress can change the client's relation to her therapist and may motivate what seem to be primitive or less organized behaviors—responses that others may label as deterioration or decompensation. Such reactions may lead the clinician to question the further use of exploratory or abuse-focused therapy with such a fragile or problematic individual.

Initially the therapist's task seemed clear: to foster increased awareness, processing, and integration of child abuse experiences by assisting in the resolution of abuse-related trauma. However, as she is confronted with the potential fruits of this recapitulation—client rage, regression, increased intrusive symptoms, and so forth—the therapist may feel that she has gone too far: somehow instigated a potential catastrophe by opening the Pandora's box of her client's past. Unfortunately, because many mental health professionals (especially in the current zeitgeist) do not want to know about sexual abuse or believe that such material should be avoided whenever possible, the clinician's peers or supervisors may reinforce her greatest fears: that she has gone somewhere that she should not have.

This chapter presents a different perspective. It acknowledges that, as described in chapter 7, severe childhood victimization is often experienced by the adult survivor as "chunks" of relatively unintegrated, avoided, often dissociated pain and dysphoria, which nevertheless exerts a strong, albeit unconscious, negative influence over her adult functioning. Given the client's denial and dissociative defenses, it is assumed that therapy must necessarily work to bring such material gradually into the open, where the client can view, process, and eventually integrate it into adult awareness. This process of therapeutically replaying previously avoided abuse material, however, may release a gestalt of archaic feelings and thoughts and a proclivity for seemingly regressed behavior. These often egodystonic reactions may frighten the adult client and, in some instances, his or her therapist. Fortunately, if done well, with sensitivity, and at the correct pace, abuse-focused therapy can take advantage of these responses, work directly with previously unavailable states, and assist in the development of a more whole and less distressed individual.

The solution to having the "tiger by the tail" is, therefore, to hang on, to stay with the client until she is through with what she has to do—no matter how uncomfortable the ride may be for the therapist. In contrast, it is likely that a therapeutic approach that fosters the client's continued avoidance of abuse-related affects and memories, or only superficially addresses them, will not result in significant improvement.

ABUSE CHARACTERISTICS AND
TREATMENT-RELATED "DETERIORATION"

In a chapter such as this one, where severe abuse-related problems are discussed, it is important to restate that not all sexual abuse victims sustain major long-term trauma, and that of those whose abuse-related problems persist into adulthood, not all present with severe personal or interpersonal difficulties. Given this variability, we may also assume that not every sexual abuse survivor in therapy will "get worse before she gets better." What, then, determines whether an individual in treatment will progress fairly evenly, with, perhaps, only minor setbacks or brief periods of increased dysphoria, or, instead, despite what is often an initial facade of relative psychological health, will experience significant psychological disturbance before further improvement?

Although, as noted in previous chapters, the complexities of child maltreatment make it difficult to know what exactly is traumagenic and what is not, certain characteristics of the original abuse experience nevertheless appear to affect client response to abuse-related therapy. In this regard, we may ask what aspects of sexual victimization produce especially high levels of denial, dissociation, and other avoidance strategies, such that integration is especially low (i.e., that the unprocessed "chunks" are especially large), and thus therapeutically revealed material appears especially intrusive and threatening.

Extreme Abuse

Clinical experience and several research studies (Briere & Conte, 1993; Herman & Schatzow, 1987) suggest that the adult whose childhood included especially severe abuse is more likely to avoid complete conscious access to such events and may respond more extremely to therapeutic restimulation of these memories. Among the characteristics of abuse that motivate extreme avoidance may be early onset and extended duration; incest, especially at the hands of a parent or parent-figure; use of physical violence by the abuser (e.g., physically forced intercourse, concurrent beatings); multiple perpetrators, either within the family (e.g., instances where both parents or multiple generations molest the child) or in "sex rings" (Burgess & Grant, 1988); and more intrusive acts (e.g., oral, anal, or vaginal penetration).

As suggested by several authors (e.g., Elliott & Briere, 1995), however, the extent to which such abuse characteristics are perceived as requiring the use of avoidance is as much a function of the survivor's internal capacities to deal with such trauma as it is the amount of trauma. Thus, although the previously noted forms of severe abuse may increase the likelihood of extreme distress, those individuals with sufficient internal coping strategies or self-capacities may nevertheless circumvent the need for defenses as primitive as extreme denial or extensive dissociation. These individuals, although often somewhat posttraumatic, often do not exacerbate as significantly on exposure to abuse-related affects or cognitions.

Concurrent Psychological Abuse or Neglect

As traumatic as sexual abuse may be, these effects may be intensified and augmented by psychological and emotional maltreatment. Chronic verbal punitiveness, frequent criticisms and insults, emotional neglect, and other forms of nonphysical abuse produce their own long-term effects (Briere & Runtz, 1988b; Demaré & Briere, 1994; Hart & Brassard, 1987) and appear to have specific impacts on children's reactions to concurrent sexual victimization.

By conveying to the child that he or she is bad or worthless, such maltreatment increases the victim's sense of having deserved the molestation and of not having warranted any better form of treatment. These and similar messages increase the victim's sense of shame and guilt at having been abused and underlie her perception of maltreatment as an appropriate response to her "badness"—conclusions that may motivate reduced conscious contact with such molestation experiences. This desire to avoid awareness of sexual abuse may be especially high if the victim was, in fact, punished or threatened for disclosing abuse or for expressing abuse-related pain. I have, for example, encountered several clients who were beaten for telling others of their abuse or who were forced to engage in painful or humiliating activities (e.g., holding Tabasco sauce in one's mouth, eating soap, or kneeling on bottlecaps for hours) as punishment for crying, resisting, or trying to escape during or after sexual molestation. This concomitant emotional maltreatment not only interferes with the development of self-capacities in the young child, as noted earlier in this book, but also tends to amplify the effects of sexual abuse by producing cognitive distortions (e.g., guilt or shame) regarding the victim's deservingness abusive treatment.

Pseudoparticipation

In a significant proportion of cases victims of sexual abuse are groomed, trained, or forced by their perpetrators to initiate or respond to sexual behaviors. This may range from being told to ask for sexual contact or to respond to sexual abuse with expressions of pleasure, to being taught to "seduce" the abuser or others (e.g., siblings or friends). Some perpetrators, in fact, have been known to devote considerable attention to sexually arousing their victims so that, in the words of one molester, "She's tied to me forever by her own feelings of pleasure; she becomes part of it too." After repeated experiences of this kind, some children become prematurely sexualized—actually seeking out sexual contact and in some instances deriving physical pleasure from it.

Although such behaviors are still clearly abusive, regardless of the child's eventual "participation" or response, adults with backgrounds of pseudoparticipation are prone to feelings of extreme guilt and responsibility (e.g., Sgroi & Bunk, 1988). During psychotherapy, nondissociated access to these experiences may be difficult, as the survivor seeks to avoid not only the memories themselves but also intense feelings of shame and self-blame. Additionally, the therapist's comments vis-à-vis the perpetrator may come to be consciously or unconsciously understood by the survivor as statements about herself because she believes that she shares the blame for the abuse.

Ongoing Abuse

When a young adult presents to a psychotherapist with issues involving childhood sexual abuse, it is frequently assumed that the victimization itself is in the past. Unfortunately, for some adults (e.g., approximately 10% of the author's lifetime survivor caseload) and a larger group of older adolescents, the victim is still sexually involved with at least one of her perpetrators. In many cases, this situation involves the client's father or stepfather, or a family friend who has become the client's "sugar-daddy." In most instances, the survivor initially keeps this relationship from the therapist, feeling ashamed and fearing rejection or ridicule. This secret can be destructive, however, as the survivor's guilt escalates and as she continues to withhold the fact of her continuing sexual contact with the abuser from her therapist.

Ongoing abuse stimulates avoidance and nonintegration of earlier molestation for several reasons. First, abuse memories may be even more threatening for the ongoing victim than for others because they remind her of her current, extremely guilt-inducing situation and emphasize its abusive and exploitive basis. Second, the client's ongoing relationship with the abuser may, in her mind, retroactively imply earlier participation and consent, and thus the client's normal anger toward her perpetrator may be turned toward herself. Finally, given the level of avoidance she must marshal to overlook or tolerate her ongoing/current abuse, the survivor may become extensively involved in denial and numbing, producing a brittle facade that is highly easily threatened by awareness-building interventions of any kind.

Sadistic and "Ritualistic" Abuse

Because of all types of sexual abuse this last form is least often described and most distressing to hear, sadistic abuse has only recently been understood to any extent by therapists. Nevertheless, it is now becoming clear that this especially malignant type of victimization is considerably more frequent than previously thought (Salter, 1995), and that the terror, horror, and pain associated with such acts may cause them to be dissociated quickly and completely by the victim.

Sadistic abuse refers to acts engaged in against a child by an adult who derives sexual pleasure by inflicting pain or degradation. Examples of such sexual torture are burning and mutilation during a sexual assault (including cutting of genitals and nipples, beating of the child during rape, use of electrical drills or surgical instruments, etc.); insertion of dirt, feces, insects, or various other objects into the vagina or anus; and the victim being tied, restrained, or bound for extended periods of time during which various sexual acts are performed. A critical component of such acts is the perpetrator's enjoyment of the victim's pain and distress, a response that is often apparent to the victim.

Ritualistic abuse differs from sadistic abuse in that the former is thought to be done in the context of an organized group and involves more ritualized behaviors rather than being solely for sadosexual pleasure. Self-reported survivors of this form of abuse often describe various rites by multiple perpetrators, wherein the child victim is part of a ceremony involving repeat victimization, especially abhorrent acts, and sexual debasement.

As noted by Kelley (1996) and others, it is not clear what proportion of ritualistic abuse reports represent accurate descriptions of real occurrences, and what proportion may reflect distortion or confabulation associated with the extreme effects of other negative childhood experiences. Some therapists who are convinced of the presence of ritualistic abuse may also pressure susceptible clients into believing that they experienced events that may not have happened. As noted in the previous chapter, such therapist behavior is entirely inappropriate, and only serves to confuse and mislead the treatment of people with real difficulties, abuse-related or otherwise.

It is clear, however, that violent, multiperpetrator, sadistic abuse does occur and that some unknown proportion of abuse survivors have undergone childhood torture of almost incomprehensible dimension. Such acts are seemingly good candidates for partial, if not complete, dissociative amnesia in some individuals. In addition, reports of these acts are so difficult for others to accept that some victims of childhood torture are disbelieved by therapists and nontherapists alike: seemingly an instance wherein dissociation extends to the social system.

Impact on the Psychotherapeutic Process

In combination or separately, these various intensifiers of abuse trauma often have a twofold effect: (a) If early enough and severe enough, they preclude the development of adequate self-capacities that might otherwise allow greater processing of distress; and (b) by virtue of their extremity, they may cause the survivor to especially avoid aspects of the internal and external environment that trigger painful memories. As noted in chapter 7, the survivor thus finds herself in a double bind: Therapy that may eventually offer relief from the frightening and painful abuse-related symptoms also involves, by nature, the recapitulation of childhood trauma she seeks to avoid. Viewed from this perspective, we must appreciate the bravery entailed in being a psychotherapy client for such individuals. Further, we may then understand the "extreme" or "abnormal" reactions to therapy that frequently arise from this dilemma. Presented subsequently are several of the most problematic of these responses.

Heightened Transference

Transference, as described in chapter 5, involves client reactions to his or her therapist that are projections of earlier experiences with significant others in the client's life. As was also noted because the abuse survivor's childhood was generally aversive, such transference is likely to be negative or at least highly ambivalent—producing angry, fearful, or stereotypically sexualized responses to potentially neutral clinician behavior or stimuli. These responses, if not handled appropriately, may impede the process of treatment, as well as potentially stimulating negative countertransference in the psychologically vulnerable therapist.

Severe sexual abuse may produce more transferential intrusion than otherwise would be expected, an outcome that, in turn, can easily result in escalating difficulties as treatment progresses. The client with a history of extreme maltreatment may be especially unable to integrate her childhood trauma with adult awareness, given the high levels of denial and dissociation she has necessarily had to invoke. For this reason her responses to replaying these experiences in therapy may be especially archaic and childhood specific. To the extent that the client thus may briefly "become" the abused child at points in therapy, the therapist is proportionately more likely to be seen as a parent or abuser.

The frequent effect of this involuntary return to childhood is a highly ambivalent, emotionally intense client-therapist relationship, where transferential affect and "acting out" or tension reduction is especially common. Typical responses include periods of objectively unwarranted rage at the therapist for imagined or minor sins; cycles of idealization and devaluation; excessive need for approval, with concurrent expectations of rejection; overattachment and, in some cases, intrusion into the therapist's personal life; adversariality, manifesting as manipulativeness; and intrusive sexualization of the therapeutic relationship.

Self-Harm

The sexual abuse survivor's tendency to turn anger and self-hatred into self-injurious acts is described throughout this book. As presented in chapters 1 through 3, this self-harm often occurs during periods of abuse-related dysphoria, when depression, self-blaming thoughts, and inwardly directed anger are especially prominent. It should not be surprising, then, that the resurgence of especially humiliating or shameful memories and feelings may also stimulate some survivors' potential for harmful tension-reduction behaviors, especially if denial and dissociation had previously been high or the therapeutic window has been exceeded. In this regard, the need to reduce especially angry or shame-related internal states motivates tension-reduction activities that are potentially more self-injurious than otherwise might be the case.

At the most immediate level, this tension reduction may manifest as dissociated, seemingly reflexive, minor self-injury during the psychotherapy session. Examples of such low-level self-mutilation include self-distracted scratching of one's hands, arms, or chest while discussing stressful material; clawing at one's scalp or neck; hitting one's head or fists against a nearby wall; or poking at oneself with objects, such as pencils or paperclips. On other occasions, however, the need for self-injurious behavior may peak minutes or hours after emotionally intense sessions, especially if previously avoided or dissociated memories were processed.

A common scenario in this regard is presented subsequently, as we consider a client described in earlier chapters.

As the reader will recall, Alice is a young woman who had recently been admitted to a psychiatric hospital for her third time, during a severe dissociative reaction. She has a long history of self-mutilatory episodes, as well as a total of five suicide attempts. Although Alice was not forthcoming about childhood victimization, her roommate reports that Alice, her younger sister, and (later) a friend were repeatedly sexually abused by her father more than 4 consecutive years, until his eventual imprisonment (her sister contracted syphilis and child welfare authorities were notified).

After Alice is discharged from the hospital, outpatient appointments are arranged. Fortuitously, one of the nurses on Alice's unit is aware of the implications of sexual abuse trauma and ensures that Alice's outpatient therapist has experience with abuse survivors. Alice is very reluctant to talk about her past. Using an approach similar to that advocated in earlier chapters, the clinician slowly and gently facilitates access to and partial processing of Alice's abuse-related affective responses and abuse memories, and works to counter Alice's pervasive self-blaming cognitions.

During her 37th session, Alice develops a powerful flashback, reexperiencing an occasion when her father forced her to have oral–genital contact with her sister. She becomes highly agitated and distraught, but slowly calms as her therapist places the event in context, engages in consolidation interventions, and applauds her progress. Because of the power and disruptiveness of this flashback, however, her therapist schedules another session for 2 days hence, elicits Alice's evaluation of her psychological state, and reminds her of several self-control techniques (e.g., calling friends or exercising) that she had used in the past to counter self-mutilatory impulses.

Alice does not appear for her next appointment, and her therapist is later contacted by an emergency room physician. He reports that Alice has made a suicide "gesture," involving ingestion of approximately 10 of her mother's low-dose tranquilizers. On discharge from the emergency room, Alice attends a session with her therapist and describes the hours after their last session. After leaving the office, she had "wandered around downtown" in a seemingly dissociated state for several hours. She states that "The next thing I knew, I was with Andy [an abusive ex-boyfriend] in his apartment," smoking crack cocaine. She relates having sex with Andy's friend, crying, and calling him names during and after intercourse, and then somehow returning to the streets, "all the time with bad thoughts running through my mind." She has no memory of how she later ended up at her mother's house ("I don't even like her") or of taking her mother's pills.

Alice continues in therapy and slowly recovers further memory fragments and "little kid" feelings, although never again at the intensity of her earlier experience. The following 6 months of treatment were difficult, however, marked by periods of depression, unfocused anger, and two more cocaine binges, along with a temporary return to her ex-boyfriend Andy and his friend.

Many aspects of Alice's story typify the incursion of self-injurious impulses into abuse-oriented therapy. First, although her current behavior occurred within the context of psychotherapy, the tension-reduction and avoidance activities she engaged in were ones she had used many times in the past. Second, her acute episode of self-injury was anteceded by an intrusive abuse-specific memory and escalating negative affect, as opposed to merely happening "out of the blue." Third, much of her behavior occurred during a dissociative episode, as is often the case when the survivor is struggling to somehow titrate unwanted awareness (i.e., her forced sexual contact with her sister). Finally, Alice's self-injurious behaviors were those frequently seen in abuse-related "acting out": suicidality (of low lethality in this case); substance abuse (the substances of choice usually being alcohol and stimulants, such as cocaine or amphetamines); and seemingly indiscriminate but, in actuality, sometimes specifically degrading or hurtful sexual behavior. Also sometimes present is self-mutilation, although in Alice's case there may not have been the time or the opportunity for this behavior, which usually occurs when the survivor is alone and after some rumination.

Not a major factor in Alice's case, except perhaps in terms of her low lethality suicide attempt, is a last quality of some abuse-related self-harm: self-injury as a method of communicating with or influencing one's therapist. Thus, as noted in chapters 1 and 3, suicide attempts or self-mutilation can be a form of interpersonal behavior for some survivors, allowing them to say or demand things that they believe cannot otherwise be said or asked for (Gil & Briere, 1995; Runtz & Briere, 1986). For instance, Alice's suicide attempt may have been, in part, a way to tell her therapist about how much abuse memories hurt and how bad she feels, or to punish the clinician's exploration of abuse material so that it would not happen again.

"Deterioration"

In addition to those behaviors that are manifestly self-injurious, some survivors more generally appear to "get worse" at points in abuse-focused therapy. As noted earlier, such seeming deterioration may suggest to the clinician (or it may be suggested to her) that uncovering treatment is contraindicated or that the therapist is mismanaging treatment. In some cases, such feedback is accurate. There are times when exploratory or processing interventions are inappropriate, for example, with highly unstable individuals (especially those with grossly inadequate self-capacities), or during periods of extreme stress or crisis. Under such circumstances, the therapist may commit process errors by moving too fast, exposing the client to potentially overwhelming material, unduly confronting survivor defenses, or otherwise exceeding the therapeutic window. In other instances, however, an increase in symptoms or dysphoria may arise as a logical effect of treatment-related decreases in dissociation and other avoidant responses.

As described earlier, the process of confronting, processing, and integrating long-avoided memories implies, at minimum, psychological discomfort. Dissociation and denial serve as defenses against the painful affect that would otherwise accompany full awareness. Thus, fuller recall of dissociated material must necessarily include a resurgence of distress, although usually not at its original intensity. The most frequently reported problems that arise during abuse-oriented therapy are increased anxiety and "new" PTSD reactions.

The anxiety reactions most commonly associated with increased access to previously avoided abuse material appear to be free-floating anxiety, fearful preoccupation, and panic attacks. "Free-floating anxiety," present in many abuse survivors to some extent, refers to a general sense of fearfulness that cannot be pinned down to any one cause. This reaction may be substantial for the individual whose unconscious awareness of abuse issues has been restimulated by psychotherapy or other abuse-relevant events. Such fear-fulness is often experienced as free floating because the relevant material is still partially dissociated, denied, or cognitively avoided, and thus the survivor is unclear as to why, in fact, he or she is so anxious. In addition, the process of psychotherapy is diffusely threatening because it implies potential for further awareness of aversive events.

In addition to free-floating anxiety, abuse-focused therapy may restimulate the survivor's childhood experience of lack of control. This sense of helplessness often emerges in the form of panic attacks: sudden episodes of intense fear that escalate as a function of their intrusiveness and seeming uncontrollability. As many individuals with such episodes will attest, one of the most powerful precipitants of panic attacks is the growing fear that another one will occur. From the survivor's perspective, this process may develop as follows: (a) the emergence of abuse-related memories, feelings, or responses during therapy is frightening, both in terms of their unpredictabil-ity and their actual content; (b) along with concomitant free-float-ing anxiety, this intense fear of one's own thoughts and affects is itself seen as further evidence of loss of control; leading to (c) an escalating spiral of fear stimulating fear, panic attacks, and other extreme anxiety states.

As has been noted in chapters 1 and 3, survivors of sexual abuse are especially prone to depression, as well as anxiety. This tendency to respond to stress with dysthymic mood may be exacerbated dur-ing psychotherapy, where the survivor's usual defenses against abuse-related dysphoria may be lessened. As she comes to confront the full extent of her victimization, and more fully experience its results, the psychic pain that accrues from such awareness typically becomes more obvious. As a result, the client in abuse-focused ther-apy may report periods of increased dejection, isolation, neediness, or hopelessness.

Finally, psychotherapy of abuse trauma may trigger, in some indi-viduals, a resurgence of PTSD-like reactions, including increased flashbacks, dissociative episodes, nightmares, and sleep disturbance (see Elliott & Briere, 1995, for an empirical study of this phenome-non). This is undoubtedly because, just as PTSD symptoms can be restimulated by similar events in the posttraumatic environment, abuse-related problems often intensify when therapy "reminds" the client of childhood victimization. These restimulations, in turn, can produce intense emotional or physical reactions during treatment, such as panic attacks, intense self-disgust, waves of nausea, or sudden headaches, most of which terminate when the session ends or the focus of discussion changes.

Together these various therapy-associated experiences may engender a crisis of faith for the client, whose initial fears regarding psychotherapy and self-examination may appear to have been justified. Fortunately, this resurgence of posttraumatic distress is not always extreme, and most typically recedes over the course of treatment. The rate at which this remission occurs is a function of the extent and severity of the original abuse trauma, as well as the pace of therapy and the extent of the client's current psychological resources.

Although the survivor of severe abuse may temporarily feel worse, she is often also aware of simultaneously feeling stronger. This latter experience may derive from two related processes. First, the lessened need to avoid one's abuse appears to free up emotional and psychological energy otherwise involved in active avoidance, allowing greater awareness, free attention, and interaction with the "here and now." Second, the experience of confronting one's greatest fears and yet of not being annihilated can foster a growing sense of mastery and self-efficacy. As a 27-year-old woman with a history of severe sibling sexual abuse concluded, "It's true that I'm having a bad time these days, but I've never been so alive, either."

Treatment Implications

The treatment implications of "teasing the dragon" are several. Perhaps most important, the potential for abuse-focused treatment to especially exacerbate the symptomatology of some severely abused individuals must be closely monitored. Although this process can reflect the positive effects of treatment, it must be evaluated constantly for its possible destabilizing effects. Destabilization, wherein the client is substantially less able to function in the outside world by virtue of uncontrollable internal experience, is *not* an acceptable effect of therapy, although it may occur in a minority of instances despite effective intervention. As opposed to the moderate and temporary exacerbation of symptoms and distress, destabilization indicates that the survivor is becoming chronically overwhelmed by the material—that exposure to traumatic affects, sensations, and cognitions has exceeded the survivor's internal capacities to "handle" them adequately. This temporary decompensation may easily increase client dependency on the therapist by virtue of her increased debility, stigmatize her by producing more florid symptoms and upsetting experiences, and deprive her of the experience of growing internal control—thereby reinforcing abuse-related schema involving helplessness and hopelessness.

At the clinical level, treatment-related destabilization indicates that the therapeutic window has been exceeded. This overstimulation may occur as a result of therapist error, or arise spontaneously because of extratherapeutic events (e.g., environmental triggers) that occur during the therapy period. In response, the therapist should immediately institute consolidating, supporting, and soothing interventions, as opposed to further exploratory or evocatory ones. Although destabilization may be unavoidable in some instances (e.g., when the survivor adds to appropriate therapeutic exposure via outside reading or support groups, or experiences major conflicts in his or her occupation or relationships), the therapeutic goal is to return the client to a state of greater internal control and stability as soon as possible. The overbridging concern is the client's safety and dignity—providing structure and support up to and including the unlikely possibility of brief psychiatric hospitalization, if necessary.

Conversely, the process of "getting worse before you get better" is often a natural one, which should not be overdramatized or pathologized. When the client describes an increase in anxiety, depression, or posttraumatic stress arising from the work that does not exceed the therapeutic window (and therefore does not destabilize), it is important for the clinician to not catastrophize the client's difficulties. The therapist who is unprepared for exacerbation may easily overreact to increased symptomatology by invoking heroic—albeit potentially unnecessary—interventions that can retraumatize the survivor and precipitate further difficulties. In the therapist's attempt to protect all involved, including, perhaps, herself vis-à-vis a civil suit, the client's confidentiality may be violated, psychiatric medications may be started or increased, and hospital-ization may be initiated. Although each of these options has its place, they are all potentially stigmatizing if mishandled, and may easily communicate to the client that he is sick, out of control, and getting worse.

There appear to be, in fact, a small subset of abuse survivors who have unnecessarily become chronic psychiatric patients. These indi-viduals may be prescribed antipsychotic medications and are often frequently hospitalized with diagnoses, such as schizophrenia, major depression with psychotic features, or atypical psychosis (Beck & van der Kolk, 1987, cited in van der Kolk, 1987). Although the lives of such individuals are chaotic and fragmented, they often cling tightly to their psychiatric role and identity—choosing (in the absence of helpful, long-term psychotherapy) sedating drugs and highly structured, controlling environments over living with abuse-related pain. The clinician who overreacts to client "deterioration" with inappropriate medication or hospitalization may find a will-ing partner in some abuse survivors, who have learned to rely on immediate—but temporary—medical/psychiatric solutions to oth-erwise aversive psychological states.

In contrast to some clinicians' overreaction to client distress, other therapists unconsciously use the exact opposite defense when con-fronted with escalating dysphoria or disorganization: They deny any evidence that the survivor is in unusual pain or experiencing greater psychological difficulties. As a result, such clinicians often fail to moderate the pace or intensity of treatment downwardly, despite their client's obvious increased distress. Although the motive for this unresponsiveness is usually benign (i.e., the therapist's anx-iety that the client may, in fact, be "getting worse"), it is frequently perceived by the survivor as abandonment ("You don't care how I feel, just like my father/mother/uncle didn't") or incompetence ("You don't know what is happening to me—you're not in control of this process"), either of which may stimulate further dysphoria and "decompensation."

This last scenario illustrates a final point regarding therapy-based increases in client disturbance: Although helpful treatment does not overemphasize the survivor's pathology or underestimate her strengths, it also recognizes the psychic stress that often accompanies exploration of severe abuse trauma. Thus, the clinician must be prepared to slow the pace of treatment, provide greater structure, or use other therapeutic interventions that allow the client to remain safe and psychologically present during the especially difficult points in her therapy while, at the same time, seeing such difficult times as potential evidence of future improvement.

Group Therapy   9

The focus of this book is clearly on the basic psychotherapy dyad—client and therapist—as opposed to other types of treatment. Other forms of therapy also may be useful in work with abuse survivors, however, especially to the extent that they incorporate a broader social or interpersonal focus. For this reason, another treatment modality—group therapy—is addressed in this chapter. In the previous edition of this book, family therapy was covered in this chapter as well. It is no longer included here based on (a) the likelihood that family therapy has less relevance to the adult survivor than does group treatment and (b) the relative dearth of available information on nonsexist, non–victim-blaming approaches to abuse-focused family treatment. For information on an additional form of treatment, that of couples therapy for the survivor and her or his partner, the reader is referred to writing on this topic by Victoria Follette (1991; Follette & Pistorello, 1995).

Group therapy is often a powerful adjunct in the treatment of post-sexual-abuse trauma. Although this modality is outlined here, the reader requiring more detail is referred to the broad literature on group treatment of abuse survivors, including papers by Abbott (1995); Blake-White and Kline (1985); Cole (1985); Cole and Barney (1987); Courtois (1988); Draucker (1992); Gil (1988); Goodman and Nowak-Scibelli (1985); Gordy (1983), Herman (1992); Herman and

Schatzow (1984); Lubell and Soong (1982); NiCarthy, Merriam, and Coffman, (1984); and Paddison, Einbinder, Maker, and Strain (1993).

As most of the preceding authors note, group therapy has certain advantages over individual psychotherapy alone. These include the benefits of lessened isolation and stigmatization, reduced shame, the development of early interpersonal trust, and identification with a supportive network of other, similarly injured individuals. Additionally, participation in such groups offers the survivor the opportunity to help as well as to be helped—a process that supports self-esteem and lessens the sense of being a deviant, passive recipient of treatment.

Although there are many principles that apply to group therapy with any client population (Yalom, 1975), certain issues and parameters are especially relevant to work with survivors of severe sexual victimization. The most important of these are outlined subsequently.

SCREENING

Because of the variable psychological functioning found among sexual abuse survivors, most therapy group leaders require that prospective members attend a pregroup evaluation interview. This meeting allows the group leaders to assess the client's level of psychological disturbance, and her or his ability to withstand the stress of group treatment. The philosophy of this screening process is perhaps best articulated by Cole and Barney (1987):

> The screening interview includes a reciprocal exchange of information. Emphasis is placed on the fact that both therapist and potential group member must make a decision about the interviewee's participation in the group. Thus the survivor's ability to be a part of the decision-making process and act on her own behalf is underscored as is the therapist's responsibility to set limits and "do no harm." The prominent themes in a survivor's life, taking care of oneself and appropriate (or inappropriate) exercise of responsibility by authority figures, are relevant even in this early context. (p. 603)

Although the minimal criteria for group participation varies from therapist to therapist (Tsai & Wagner, for example, advocate accepting "all women who report a molestation experience and wish to participate in a group" [1978, p. 426], as do NiCarthy et al. [1984]), many workers in this area suggest screening out individuals who are (a) either chronically unstable or currently in crisis, (b) currently abusing drugs or alcohol, (c) psychotic, or (d) suicidal.

Although none of these exclusion criteria are problematic, they are surprisingly similar to the major long-term effects of sexual abuse, as described in chapters 1 through 3. Thus, if taken to their extreme, these criteria might successfully screen out most survivors of severe abuse, leaving only those with less need for treatment. For this reason the following strategy is suggested:

1. Carefully evaluate each client for the presence of the above difficulties, as well as any other relevant concerns.
2. Determine the actual extent of each problem (e.g., there may well be a considerable difference between the group functioning of a severely suicidal person versus one who has passing suicidal thoughts, or between a woman who occasionally uses recreational amounts of cocaine and a heroin addict).
3. Determine whether such negative factors, as mediated by any specific strengths (e.g., good affect regulation capacities), are likely to interfere with each particular client's individual response to group therapy. If the answer is yes, the client should be referred back to her individual therapist until a later point in time when she is more ready for the stress of a group experience. The answer may be no, however, if the prospective member is not psychotic, out of touch with reality, substance addicted, overly impulsive, or unable to interact appropriately with others. Additionally, even these problems may not rule out a survivor's participation if the group is specifically designed for such issues (e.g., a group for substance-addicted incest survivors). Thus, at least from the author's perspective, group screening criteria should be seen as important guidelines—not necessarily as rigid requirements. The ultimate question the therapist must ask herself is: Does this client have sufficient inner resources and few enough interfering factors that he or she could attend this group without becoming a casualty of the treatment process?

Perhaps more important than screening criteria is the notion of matching group members within a given group. If the group is for "borderline" abuse survivors in an inpatient setting, few of the above criteria apply. In fact, in such groups, individuals with good self-capacities would be screened out because their participation might (a) lead them to feel more dysfunctional than actually may be the case (e.g., "Am I like them?"), or (b) cause more injured group members to feel shame or implicit failure ("Why aren't I more like her or him?").

Most broadly, based on the notion of the therapeutic window outlined in chapter 6, the issue is less whether a given member is symptomatic than whether the self-capacities—and thus the "windows"—of the group members generally are in accord. For example, some survivors within a nonscreened group might have broad access to painful material (i.e., able to recall, express, and process painful material without being overwhelmed) whereas others might have more narrow access (i.e., only able to experience small amounts of distressing thoughts, feeling, or memories before becoming destabilized). In such a case, those survivors able to work at relatively intense emotional levels may inadvertently overwhelm other members for whom merely hearing such material results in excessive restimulation and causes them to significantly exceed their respective therapeutic windows. In response, some group members may escalate emotionally during the session or, even more unfortunately, be forced to "act out" (tension-reduce) after group as a way of reducing overwhelming distress.

Because of the possibility of discordant therapeutic windows producing iatrogenic outcomes for survivors with lower self-capacities (as well as guilt and distress among those whose appropriate group work was seemingly injurious to others), it is recommended that survivors be matched on their relative level of self functioning rather than the extent of their trauma. Thus, those with narrower therapeutic windows are included in groups with others at the same level of functioning, whereas those with wider windows are placed in groups where more intense material can be openly expressed and processed without negative outcome.

CONCURRENT INDIVIDUAL PSYCHOTHERAPY

As described earlier, the process of group treatment is inherently a stressful one for abuse survivors. Not only does the client have his own painful memories to disclose and to work on in front of relative strangers, he must also listen to painfully detailed accounts of other members' betrayal and victimization. The effect of these group experiences can be escalating anxiety and anger, and restimulation of abuse-related flashbacks and intrusive thoughts.

This high level of stress not only requires matching of self-capacities within a given group, careful attention to group process, and specific timing of interventions for each group member, but also suggests the need for concurrent individual psychotherapy. Of the many abuse-focused groups that I have supervised, the few negative outcomes have typically involved survivors whose internal resources have been overwhelmed by powerful group processes and who have had no external (out-of-group) therapeutic supports to call on.

Such individuals additionally often demand or elicit a disproportionate share of the group's attention and may become disruptive as a result of their compensatory interpersonal behavior. By virtue of their monopolizing the group's attention and agenda, these clients may eventually become ostracized or attacked by other group members—leading to further alienation and distress. In some cases, this "fallout" from group is clinically manageable but requires that the therapists become personally involved (Courtois & Leehan, 1982), thus violating the important group therapy maxim of "equal attention for all."

For this reason many clinicians insist that group members also have regular outside psychotherapists (Abbott, 1995; Cole & Barney, 1987; Goodman & Nowak-Scibelli, 1985; Gordy, 1983; Herman & Schatzow, 1984; Lubell & Soong, 1982). This division of labor allows the survivor to gain from the social interaction, feedback, destigmatization, and support of group psychotherapy, and yet have an individual therapist who can devote her or his full attention to the client and her more pressing needs and issues. Thus, although leaders of high functioning groups—where all suicidal, substance abusing, and "emotionally unstable" clients have been screened out—may not feel the need for a concomitant therapy rule, therapists of most abuse groups (e.g., in mental health centers, drug treatment facilities, psychiatric inpatient units, or postincarceration settings) are well advised to make this a requirement.

OTHER GROUND RULES

In addition to concomitant individual psychotherapy, it is usually a good idea to introduce a few other ground rules at the onset of group therapy. The most common of these are as follows:

1. *Attendance.* Members should try to attend every session of the group, especially if it is closed or short term. It is often further requested that if a member is considering dropping out of group, that he or she return at least one last time to share that decision with the group.
2. *Confidentiality.* Participants are asked to refrain from discussing the group with nonmembers, both in terms of the material disclosed during sessions and the identities of the group participants.
3. *Outside contact.* Some clinicians (Goodman & Nowak-Scibelli, 1985) request that participants not socialize outside of group meetings, whereas others (Herman & Schatzow, 1984) place no constraints on outside contact. The argument in favor of noncontact is that the neediness and interpersonal disturbance of some abuse survivors can produce occasional intense and disruptive interactions or boundary violations outside of group, where they cannot be controlled by the group leaders. Such interactions, in addition to being potentially injurious to the members involved, may also have negative impacts on the group's functioning. Examples of such behaviors are clients who make repetitive and unwanted phone calls or visits to other group members, members attempting to coerce other members into sexual contact, and subgroups of members having "councils of war" regarding disliked other members. Although I do not advocate a no-contact rule per se (among other things, such rules are virtually unenforceable and frequently reinforce therapist-client power dynamics), it is recommended that clients be asked to forego sexual relationships with other group members, at least during the tenure of the group, and that, most important, any significant contacts between group members that occur outside of group be brought into the next session where they can be discussed.
4. *"Air time."* A final recommended ground rule is that all group members be allowed a certain amount of uninterrupted time per session to speak about their issues, concerns, or feelings. This may be ensured by having all members begin each session with a brief presentation of how their week went, how they are feeling presently, and other relevant material. Other groups have a "no-interruption" rule, whereby

any member is deemed to have the right to speak without being cut off by another member—an approach that, although egalitarian, may be abused by some especially needy, boundary-impaired, or long-winded members. Finally, in groups where the leaders take an active role, the clinician may specifically keep track of who has or has not spoken in a given session and may ask silent members if there is anything that they wish to discuss. Regardless of how this rule is enforced, the bottom line should be that all members have the right to speak—that silence is no longer being forced on them, and that the group cares that they have a chance to participate. A corollary to this notion is the reverse: that no member be coerced or pressured to speak in any given instance.

GROUP COMPOSITION

Although it is clear that abuse groups should consist of only males or only females and should usually be run by clinicians of the same gender as the members (Cole, 1985; Draucker, 1992), most other mixtures of clients (beyond the "window matching" issues described earlier) seem to work equally well together. Herman and Schatzow (1984), for example, conclude that "prospective group members' motivation and positive expectations seemed to outweigh other factors such as age, race, sexual orientation, or diagnosis in predicting a successful group outcome" (p. 3). Conversely, Paddison et al. (1993) note that "Dyads of similar background are preferred so that a member does not feel like the 'only' one (i.e., not the only member who is an African American, Hispanic, substance abuser in recovery, homosexual, married woman, single woman, mother, etc.)" (p. 38).

The only provisos that might be added to the above are that optimal group dynamics are probably most likely when (a) less verbal members are balanced by several more verbal ones, (b) one or two members are somewhat more "advanced," in the sense of having already dealt with some of their abuse issues in previous psychotherapy, and (c) the total number of participants per group ranges between 5 and 10. Regarding the last point, groups with fewer than 5 members often appear to drag or, paradoxically, become too intense, whereas groups larger than 10 often deprive individual members of needed "air time" and frequently fail to coalesce into a functioning entity.

NUMBER AND DURATION OF SESSIONS

A review of the literature on sexual abuse survivor groups reveals a considerable diversity in the number of sessions considered best for abuse survivors, although most authors agree on the length of each session (1 1/2 to 2 hours). Two writers, for example, describe group programs consisting of either 4 or 6 meetings in total (Cole, 1985; Tsai & Wagner, 1978), whereas, at the other end of the continuum, Abbott (1995), Courtois and Leehan (1982), Lubell and Soong (1982), and Paddison et al. (1993), suggest 16 to 24 sessions or more. The advantages of small numbers of sessions appear to be their economy (both in terms of time and money), their goal orientation, and the sharp focus on abuse-related issues they offer. Such groups are likely to be conceptualized as partially didactic and as serving as a prelude to other, more extensive forms of treatment (Tsai & Wagner, 1978). Longer groups, conversely, allow the members to learn about one another, to build group cohesion and a sense of trust, and to work through abuse-related interpersonal difficulties (Abbott, 1995; Courtois & Leehan, 1982).

Although the optimal number of sessions may vary according to the goals of treatment, as well as the setting in which therapy is occurring, the author has found that 10 to 12 sessions (the average number cited in the abuse group literature) is often most effective—allowing enough time for group cohesion to occur, and yet not so extended that intragroup conflicts, habitually dysfunctional behaviors, or major transference dynamics supersede or derail abuse-related concerns.

GROUP STRUCTURE

There are several basic types of group structures, different combinations of which may be adapted for work with abuse survivors. Most basically, these can be summarized as *open* versus *closed*, and *programmatic* versus *nonprogrammatic*.

Open abuse groups begin at a specific time, but continue for an indeterminate number of sessions. Because these groups are ongoing, members typically rotate in and out of them as needed. One client, for example, may enter the group at session 7, stay for the next 10 sessions, and then leave, whereas the next client might enter at session 9 and stay until session 35. The advantages of such groups include (a) their flexibility of membership, making them ideal for psychiatric hospitals or some residential settings where clients enter treatment at different times and (b) the opportunity for newer members to learn from older ones who are familiar with the group process, and who can provide helpful information and feedback.

Although open groups have several positive attributes, some survivors (especially those with issues around security, stability, and predictability) are unsettled by the shifting membership of such groups and may report never feeling entirely safe. A commonly expressed concern is that open groups do not foster a sense of community, where survivors can grow to know and count upon each other. Closed groups, conversely, do offer this opportunity for group cohesion. Such groups begin and end with most of the same members, usually after a predetermined number of sessions. Understanding and trust between group members thus becomes a major issue, as does heightened communication. Successful groups of this sort can take on a life of their own in many instances and may become central support systems for their members. Despite these obvious advantages, however closed groups also have several potential weaknesses, including the effects of client dropout over time (in most instances one or more members leave prior to the official end of group) and the duress of "waiting lists" for survivors who were not present at the beginning of the group but who nevertheless would benefit from immediate group therapy (Blake-White & Kline, 1985; Cole & Barney, 1987).

Programmatic groups proceed according to a predetermined plan, wherein each session has a specific focus and in some cases specific exercises. These groups are almost always closed and tend to be shorter than nonprogrammatic ones. Cole (1985) and Tsai and Wagner (1978), for example, list the goals and activities of each of the four to six sessions of their groups, and Herman and Schatzow (1984) have specific instructions for sessions 1, 2 to 5, 6 to 9, and 10. Most programmatic groups observe some version of the following schema: Early sessions focus on introductions, description of ground rules, didactic information on sexual abuse (both orally presented and in the form of reading lists or handouts), summary disclosures of molestation, and the development of group cohesion and identity; middle sessions are devoted to extensive discussions of individual group members' molestation experiences, with support and feedback from other members and the group leaders; and final sessions work to develop a sense of closure on the experience, including the sometimes difficult work of termination.

Nonprogrammatic groups, although usually remaining structured in terms of specific starting and stopping times, "air time" limits for each participant, and occasional prescribed homework assignments (Courtois & Leehan, 1982), nevertheless, are less subject to strictures regarding the appropriate content of any given session. The topics of each meeting are more typically determined by the participants, given the overriding assumption that the general context will still be members' abuse experiences and their ramifications. Most open groups are, of necessity, nonprogrammatic ones because it would be inappropriate for new members to enter a group halfway through a programmed series of sessions. Some long-term closed groups, however, are also nonprogrammed, especially if one of the group goals is the working through of abuse-related interpersonal concerns and issues.

In my experience, both programmed and nonprogrammed groups "work"; the choice of which type to use is primarily a function of the goals of treatment, the setting in which it will occur and the time available for therapy. Short-term, closed groups usually function best in the programmed mode, whereas long-term groups, whether open or closed, are often most effective if the agenda for each session is participant determined.

SESSION STRUCTURE

In addition to its structure across meetings, the abuse group also has form within sessions. Most groups begin with each member speaking briefly about his or her life since the last session, and about how he or she is feeling at the present moment. This activity gives each member a structured opportunity to share with the group, as well as allowing the group leaders to ascertain who may need special attention. After this exercise is completed, the group typically moves on to whatever discussions have been planned (in programmatic groups) or are generated by the participants' opening presentations (in nonprogrammatic ones). At the end of each session, the group process is recapped by the members or the leaders: Significant points are reemphasized and a more global perspective on the group's process is offered, usually stressing communalities of experience. Also at this time many therapists repeat the opening exercise: Each member, in turn, makes a brief statement on how the group went and how they are feeling.

The intent of these activities is twofold. First, anxiety is lessened by providing a predictable structure within each session. Participants know they will have several opportunities to speak but that the focus of the group will then move on to other speakers. The predictability of this routine reassures the participants that the process is under control and therefore more safe. Second, the internal structure of the session allows for closure, giving the members a sense of completeness. By wrapping up each session at its end, the therapists in some sense imply that the process is finished for that moment, and thus is no longer as threatening or evocative as it might otherwise be. In the words of one group member: "The wrap-up kind of closes the book until next week, so I can feel like, OK, let's move on to the next thing I have to do."

In contrast, a session where intense disclosures continue until the allocated amount of time runs out, at which time all members unceremoniously depart, is likely to remain anxiety provoking well beyond the end of the session. This anxiety continues partially because there has been no "official" end or closure to the experience, and there is seemingly no one to rely upon to keep it constrained and safe. Such poorly structured groups encourage tension reduction ("acting out") or other avoidance responses between sessions, as group members attempt to control their dysphoria by any means possible.

TERMINATION ISSUES

As was noted in chapter 3, many sexual abuse survivors have experienced lives dominated by abandonment and maltreatment, leading them to become hypersensitive to these issues later in life. It is, therefore, understandable that, for some individuals, termination of group therapy can be a major stressor (Abbott, 1995). The very aspects of group that are most attractive to the survivor, for example, a supportive network of understanding people and the opportunity to discuss issues intensely meaningful but difficult to share with nonabused individuals, become the most hurtful as they are seemingly taken away as group ends.

For this reason termination issues are best introduced well before the end of group therapy, just as the "last day" should be known to all from the outset of treatment. Additionally, most groups devote the last one or two sessions to discussions of what was gained by the members, "where do we go from here," and good-bye saying. Some group leaders (Herman & Schatzow, 1984) further suggest that members make a small list of people they can call on for further support after the end of group, in addition to their regular outside psychotherapists. Other, open-ended groups simply remind the terminating member that the group is ongoing and that she can "drop in, visit, and report her progress" whenever necessary (Blake-White & Kline, 1985, p. 402).

Finally, as Gordy suggests (1983), the group may decide to have a reunion session several months after the termination of group, thereby lessening the members' sense of immediate loss. Regardless of what interventions are used to deal with termination issues, however, three principles are usually present: (a) an ending date is specified well in advance, at least for closed groups; (b) frequent reminders that group participation is for a finite period of time are built into the group process, so that members may prepare themselves well in advance; and (c) the last sessions of group are "ceremonialized" (Herman & Schatzow, 1984), including devoting considerable time for leave-taking, thereby providing closure on the experience.

CONCLUSION

This brief chapter provides an overview of the principles and parameters of group treatment as they apply to sexual abuse survivors. Although group therapy, alone, is rarely sufficient for the more severely abused survivor, it can provide important experiences that are not typically available in individual psychotherapy alone. Especially impactful may be the opportunity to share previously shameful secrets with a group of people who have had similar experiences and who can offer important normalizing perspectives and experiences. Because group therapy requires the survivor to confront his or her responses to a group of people, however, it may be more threatening than individual therapy for some.

Client Gender Issues   10

Throughout this book, reference is made to both male and female sexual abuse survivors, as if the results of victimization and its ultimate treatment were similar for each sex. This approach has been intentional, based on research data and clinical experience that post–sexual-abuse trauma can manifests in comparable ways among males and females, although women generally endorse more symptoms than men. For example, the various symptom scales of the Trauma Symptom Checklist (TSC-33/40; Briere & Runtz, 1989b; Elliott & Briere, 1992) including Dissociation, Anxiety, Depression, Anger, and Sleep Disturbance, are similarly elevated among male and female sexual abuse survivors (Briere, Evans, Runtz, & Wall, 1988; Mendel, 1995; Urquiza & Crowley, 1986), as are indices of sexual dissatisfaction and poor self-concept (Urquiza & Crowley, 1986). In addition, several studies indicates that male abuse survivors may display psychological symptom patterns that are similar to those of female survivors (Hunter, 1991; Kelly, MacDonald, & Waterman, 1987; Mendel, 1995) and may produce similar MMPI profiles (Hunter, 1991).

This overlap in the ways in which males and females experience post–sexual-abuse trauma makes sense, suggesting that all humans can be hurt in similar ways by extreme stressors, regardless of gender. For example, PTSD symptoms, such as flashbacks or restimulation, occur after severe trauma in both men and women, as does postabuse depression or dissociation (Briere, 1995b). The data available in this area, therefore, support the notion that although males may retrospectively report less distress or more enjoyment of molestation at the time it transpired (Finkelhor, 1979a; Maltz & Holman, 1987), may report it less frequently to others (Briere et al., 1988), and may be less likely to perceive it as abuse, they are no more immune to its negative effects than are female survivors (Mendel, 1995).

Males and females *do* tend respond somewhat differently to traumatic events, however, partially as a result of social training to behave in sex-role appropriate ways (Bem & Lenney, 1976; Mendel, 1995; Spence & Helmreich, 1978). As these differences relate to sexual abuse, it is clear that men and women are socialized differently with regard to sexuality and aggression, responses to victimization, and expressions of emotional pain. These variations, in turn, can impact on how the survivor deals with the effects of abuse and how she or he will respond to psychotherapy.

SEXUALITY AND AGGRESSION

Ours is a society that tends to socialize men to be sexually aggressive and women to be passive and relatively easily victimized. In fact, the very motives for sexual contact may be differ to some extent between men and women: Men are encouraged by their peers, media portrayals, and other cultural forces to use sex as a vehicle for dominance and self-assertion than are women, whereas women have been encouraged traditionally to see sex more in the context of connectedness, caring, and relationship-building than have men.

Although there is little reason to believe that such cultural prescriptions are based in major biological gender differences in sexual needs or behaviors, these disparate sex roles do reflect how people, as social beings, see male versus female sexuality. These roles, in turn, can easily affect how individuals who suffer sexually related trauma respond to such injuries. Most notably, such social messages probably have significant bearing on why females who have been sexually abused are prone to revictimization, whereas male sexual abuse survivors are more likely to become sexual abuse perpetrators.

As noted in chapter 3, some sexually abused women may come to see sex as a potentially dangerous endeavor that, nevertheless, can be used to achieve other goals otherwise less available to them. Among these other outcomes are exchange for wanted commodities such as security, limited control over powerful (typically male) others, and satisfaction of unmet needs for affection, contact, and avoidance of loneliness. Learning early in life that her sexuality is one of her most valued social commodities, some female survivors especially strive to appear sexually attractive, seductive, or otherwise desirable to men. Not only do men's responses to such activities have the effect of verifying to the survivor that she is only as good as she appears or performs sexually, they also, especially when combined with trained passivity or receptivity, place her in greater danger from predatory males in her environment.

Males who have been sexually victimized as children, conversely, have not had that experience in the context of social training to be passive, ornamental, or a sex object. Victimization can be construed as sadly congruent with the female role, whereas it is antithetic to social notions of masculinity. Instead, males are encouraged from childhood to be strong, instrumental, assertive, and aggressive—traits that are incongruent with the concept of victimization (Johanek, 1988; Mendel, 1995; Stukas-Davis, 1990). Thus, the growing boy's sense of socially defined masculinity is often undermined by his abuse because victimization implies weakness and being *done to* rather than *doing to*.

As well as social proscriptions against a male "allowing" himself to be victimized, many male survivors struggle with the fact that their sexual molestation happened at the hands of another male. The combination of weakness implied by victimization and the fact of sexual contact with another man (regardless of the victim's nonconsent) is likely to lead the male victim—and many of those around him—to believe that he is homosexual. In a society as anti-homosexual as is ours, this belief may engender panic and self-disgust beyond that associated with sexual molestation.

Whether through fears of inadequacy or homosexuality, the developing male child may strive to reaffirm the power or masculinity he believes was compromised by his abuse—potentially leading to sexual aggression against others (Briere & Conte, 1989; Rogers & Terry, 1984). As one adolescent male reported: "Some time when Thomas was doing that stuff to me, I said to myself: 'When I get older, I want to be the one who does it, not the one who gets it.'"

Thus, one result of sexual molestation may be its impact on adherence to prevailing sex roles. For some women, early sexual abuse may train and support later stereotypic femininity, sexual fantasies about being forced into sex, and greater acceptance of attitudes supportive of rape (Briere, Smiljanich, & Henschel, 1994; Corne, Briere, & Esses, 1992), reinforcing traditional notions of victimization as congruent with parts of the female role. Other parts, however, such as social expectations of sexual virtue are compromised, such that the survivor may be seen by others as "easy" or "sluttish" and as unworthy of respect.

Male victimization, conversely, violates male sex-role requirements regarding invulnerability, thereby motivating in some individuals behaviors thought to bestow masculine power, such as aggression against others (Mendel, 1995). In both cases, ultimately, the sex-role–related effects of abuse are parodies of true sexual identity—just as sexual victimization, to some extent, reflects an exaggeration of social rules regarding sexual interactions.

It also should be noted, however, that for some survivors the experience of sexual abuse may lead to *rejection* of traditional sex roles. For example, the abused male may come to associate dominance and intrusion with injustice and injury, leading him to eschew such qualities in his own life and relationships. Similarly, the female survivor may come to devalue traditional conceptualizations of feminine passivity and ornamentality because she associates such attributes with vulnerability or submission to unfair male dominance. Although such individuals may suffer from the social stigmatization and rejection that often accrues from sex-role violations, they may also gain from the greater psychological flexibility associated with less stereotypic responses (Bem & Lenney, 1976). Even this greater willingness to confront prevailing sex roles, however, does not provide complete protection from sex-role stereotypic responses (Briere, Ward, & Hartsough, 1983), leading to at least some gender-specific responses to trauma for most survivors.

GENDER-SPECIFIC REACTION TO
ABUSE-RELATED EMOTIONAL TRAUMA

As described earlier, male and female survivors often differ in both their experience and expression of abuse effects. Gender-related differences in the former (i.e., how abuse-related affect is processed) may involve sex differences in how one is trained to deal with feelings. It is likely that the effects of traditional sex-role socialization directly translate into the relative level of affect regulation skills possessed by each sex. Women in our culture are socialized to be "good at" feelings: to be able to experience and express many affective states without being perceived as weak or dysfunctional. In fact, emotional expression is probably an implicit component of positive sex-role behavior in women. As a result, women appear to have relatively higher affective competence than men in some areas; they may be more able to tolerate powerful emotional experiences without necessarily having to avoid them and to be relatively facile at regulating emotional processes.

Men in our culture, conversely, have been trained to avoid emotional pain, primarily by suppressing emotional response and by acting on the environment to reduce emotional stressors. Emotional avoidance is repackaged as bravery and stoicism: the warrior who does not cry or otherwise express pain when injured, the John Wayne–like character who doesn't get mad, but assuredly gets even. Although sex-role supports for the avoidance of emotionality in men may lead to certain socially validated traits (e.g., single-minded sense of purpose, unwillingness to be side-tracked by subjective distress, or technical competence), this same process is likely to be detrimental when it comes to emotional recovery from trauma and involvement in aggressive or destructive acts. The male who has been trained to avoid emotionality, for example, may be more likely to dissociate or cognitively avoid traumatic stress, thereby having fewer opportunities to desensitize or otherwise process emotional pain as outlined in chapter 6. As a result, some male sexual abuse survivors may fail to recover fully from abuse-related trauma, inadvertently trading continued emotional avoidance for emotional healing.

An additional effect of trained emotional avoidance in men is a relatively low ability to tolerate sustained distress without acting out. To the extent that male sex-role socialization interferes with learning how to regulate affect internally, the traumatized man may be forced to externalize his pain through tension-reduction activities. This tendency toward acting out, as opposed to processing or expressing one's trauma, applies not only to male sexual abuse survivors but also to men who have suffered physical abuse during childhood (e.g., Pollock, et al., 1990; Widom, 1989). In each case the net result may be a person who suffers considerable psychic pain but who is unable to modulate or completely process it. He may, instead, seek to reduce this internal tension by engaging in acts that distract, sooth, anesthetize, or release painful affect. Such avoidance and tension-reduction activities include substance abuse, dissociated or indiscriminate sexual acts, excessive physical activity, self-mutilation (often underestimated and underassessed in men) (Briere, Henschel, Smiljanich, & Morlan-Magallanes, 1990), and seemingly impulsive acts of aggression. Regarding the latter, the reduced affect regulation capacities associated with the male sex-role may explain, in part, the greater tendency for abuse males than abused females to aggress against others later in life.

Not only are men more likely to have learned to avoid experiencing emotional pain, most males in our society grow up learning to suppress verbal expressions of pain or distress, a process that often keeps male survivors from sharing their abuse or its effects with others, and that may delay or negate their access to psychotherapy. Women, conversely, are more likely to be reinforced for communicating their feelings to others. This expressiveness can have positive ramifications for the female abuse survivor who is more likely to feel understood during therapy, and to experience the benefits of more freely accessed emotional expression and catharsis. The "down side" of this ability to express emotionality, however, is that such women may look more distressed or dysfunctional than equivalently injured males and may, in fact, be labeled (and discounted) as "histrionic" or "overly dramatic."

IMPLICATIONS FOR RESPONSE TO THERAPY

These sex-role–related processes have implications for the survivor's behavior and reactions during abuse-oriented psychotherapy. Such gender differences relate more to the *process* of treatment, however, than to the actual techniques used. In this regard, male and female differences in expressivity, range of emotional responses, freedom to be vulnerable, and access to psychic pain can influence how issues are presented, how the client responds to them, and how the therapist-client relationship develops.

SURVIVORS WHO ARE PERPETRATORS

The first gender-related issue that impacts on psychotherapy is whether the survivor is, himself, a perpetrator. Most research indicates that males who molest are more likely to have been sexually abused as children than are nonmolesters (Gebhard, Gagnon, Pomeroy, & Christenson, 1965; Johanek, 1988; Langevin, Handy, Hook, Day, & Russon, 1985; Rokous, Carter, & Prentky, 1988). Equivalent data are more rare for females—partially because most sexual abusers are male (Finkelhor, 1979a; Runtz, 1987; Russell, 1983b; Wyatt, 1985), and partially because male survivors are more likely to externalize abuse-related distress (Briere & Conte, 1989; Smiljanich & Briere, 1993).

Because of this increased potential for (primarily, but not exclusively, male) sexual aggression, I suggest that survivors presenting for psychotherapy services be gently informed of (a) the therapist's duty to warn potential victims, both at the time of screening or at any point in which it is disclosed during therapy, and (b) his or her ethical responsibility to report to police any person who admits to being a child abuser. Further, even if the police have been informed and the molester is not incarcerated, therapists without specialized training in treating offenders should avoid working with survivors who are also perpetrators. Instead, the clinician's best option may be to refer the abusing survivor to programs that specialize in treating perpetrators—the most effective of which may also address the client's own abuse history.

The preceding constraints may appear harsh to the reader, who may correctly note that individuals whose abusiveness is partially an outgrowth of their own molestation experiences deserve treatment as much as do any other survivors. Further, he or she may point out that this policy may serve only to keep survivors from disclosing their molestation activities to receive or continue therapy. I do not disagree with either point and only note that (a) the therapist must do the best she or he can to report and confront child abuse whenever it is disclosed, and (b) therapy with individuals who are molesters is very difficult work, requiring the clinician to be both a police officer and a healer. Furthermore, in many cases, sexual abusers do not stop molesting children merely because they are in treatment unless, of course they are in prison or residents of a "closed" (locked) treatment facility.

PROCESSING OF EMOTION

Of those sex-role issues affecting response to treatment in nonperpetrators, one of the most salient is in the area of awareness and expression of emotion. As noted earlier, the female sex role tends to support emotional expression and processing, whereas the male role discourages such activities. Combined with cultural expectations that males should be tough, strong, and aggressive, and, therefore, able to resist victimization, these social forces especially encourage male survivors to avoid conscious access to their molestation and its associated traumatic effects. Even when the male survivor is able to confront his abuse history, he may be more prone to intellectualization and engage in less emotional expression of his experience. The latter phenomenon may result in, for example, someone who speaks at length on the sociocultural or psychodynamic basis of victimization but who is less able to describe the impacts of abuse on his own internal state.

The male survivor's tendency to avoid, deny, suppress, or intellectualize his abuse history has obvious effects on his ability to access or express feelings regarding his trauma. This disability, in turn, reduces the amount of emotional processing he is able to accomplish during treatment. Additionally, the male survivor's frequent choice of action over affect may result in higher levels of treatment-related tension reduction or impulsive "solutions" to longstanding problems (Smiljanich & Briere, 1993; Stukas-Davis, 1990). For these reasons the therapist working with male survivors must devote more attention to emotional issues than he or she would with the average female survivor.

Successful treatment often involves even more attention to the therapeutic window for male survivors than female ones. Because the male survivor may have less overall affect regulation capacities, with associated greater reliance on cognitive and behavioral avoidance, he may require more gentle and titrated exposure to affectively upsetting material. In this regard, his therapeutic window may be more "narrow" than an equivalently abused female survivor. Among other things, some male survivors may require, at least initially, (a) less intense discussion of abuse-related issues, (b) more brief contact with upsetting abuse memories, (c) greater normalization of (often hidden) feelings of shame, hurt, and fear regarding his abuse, along with associated feelings of rejection or abandonment, and (d) greater attention to defenses, such as dissociation, denial, intellectualization, or precipitous action. Regarding the last, the clinician should maintain continuous awareness of the fact that exceeding of the therapeutic window in male survivors may be associated with a greater risk of self- or other-injurious tension reduction behaviors.

The greater likelihood of tension reduction in male survivors is often compounded by the more easily accessed anger of some male survivors. Interestingly, because males in our society are less likely to be punished for anger or expressions of hostility, this is one emotion that the therapist typically does not have as much trouble "freeing up" in men. In fact, for certain male survivors of severe abuse, anger may become the primary emotion available for expression. Such men appear to funnel less stereotypically masculine responses, such as fear, guilt, shame, or powerlessness, into the single affect of anger, which can then be triggered by a wide variety of interpersonal stimuli to produce aggressive acts.

This conversion of pain into anger is so automatic for some men that the therapist may have to work at length to help them recognize the simultaneous presence of nonangry feelings. Furthermore, when these "weaker" emotions are brought into the survivor's awareness and are verbalized, the clinician may spend even more care approaching and normalizing them than is frequently necessary for a female survivor. Among the messages that the therapist should convey are reassurances that sadness and fear are normal responses to victimization for any person, irrespective of gender, and that emotional expression is not antithetic to true masculinity. Also, it may be suggested to such clients that anger can serve as a defense against feelings of vulnerability, and he may be encouraged to examine the "softer" feelings that reside behind his rage.

In contrast to the male experience, female abuse survivors have been trained to avoid extreme or intense anger and to focus their expression more on the less threatening affective domains of sadness of fear. We need only consider the multiple pejorative words for an angry woman in our society, in contrast to the relative absence of such words for equivalent males. Given these cultural constraints on women, the therapeutic agenda may reverse: While supporting the female survivor's expression of psychic pain, the therapist may also encourage the explicit release of otherwise suppressed anger. This does not mean that the clinician should attempt to force the client into the premature expression of angry feelings. It may be appropriate, however, for the therapist to confront the female survivor gently at times when it appears that angry responses are being inhibited or replaced with feelings more appropriate to her traditional sex role. Thus, just as the male may use anger to defend against "weaker" feelings, so may the female survivor invoke dysphoria to avoid feeling the more "aggressive" affects of anger or rage. Similarly, the stereotypic male survivor may need support to keep from externalizing his distress in tension-reduction activities, whereas the stereotypic female survivor may require assistance in learning how to deal appropriately with the outside environment to increase safety and self-efficacy.

In addition to emotional issues, male and female survivors frequently differ in their response to power or control dynamics during psychotherapy. How these issues are manifest, in turn, depends to some extent on the sex of the therapist.

POWER DYNAMICS

Male Therapist, Male Client

Power dynamics are perhaps most obvious when the therapist is male, partially because he is likely to be of the same gender as the client's perpetrator. Male survivors may attempt to go "one up" or "one down" with male therapists, according to their assessment of their own vulnerability and that of the clinician. In the "one down" mode the client may present as passive or eager to please. There is the frequent sense that the therapist is seen as a potentially dangerous father figure, who must not be challenged and who may require pacification. Although such clients may appear amenable to treatment, based on their "good" presentation, their (often hidden) distrust and anger can inhibit therapeutic progress. Unfortunately, the avoidant aspects of this pattern can reduce the opportunity for such men to process the affects and cognitions associated with a "perpetrator" transference; instead, the "one down" client's approach to dominant men may be subtly reinforced.

For this reason, trust issues should be addressed frequently with acquiescent male clients, and tentative attempts at greater self-determination should be reinforced. For example, the passive male client may be encouraged to disagree with the therapist, and the therapist may seek to be especially egalitarian with him. The messages that the clinician seeks to convey are that (a) the client is not in danger from his therapist—even if angered or provoked, (b) independence of thought and opinion are good things and will not be punished, and (c) the therapist's gender will not keep him from understanding or caring.

In contrast to the "one down" male client are those who strive to dominate interactions with their male therapist. Such clients are frequently challenging, verbally aggressive, and likely to present a front of invulnerability. These "hypermasculine" reactions usually represent compensations for fearfulness and thus reflect many of the same concerns felt by the "one down" client. Specifically, the survivor who seeks to be "one up" hopes that a threatening or disinterested demeanor will forestall therapist aggression or negative judgment, as well as, in some instances, prove to the clinician that the survivor is "still a man" despite his molestation history and involvement in therapy.

The aggression and hostility expressed by such clients also represent, however, a watered-down version of their rage against their childhood perpetrators—a process that may be a positive sign, since it implies that (a) the therapist is seen as more safe than the original abuser, and (b) the client is able to experience and process at least some related affect. It is suggested that the angry survivor, regardless of gender, is sometimes healthier than the acquiescent or passive one and thus may have a better "prognosis" in certain instances.

Treatment interventions with such clients should not punish challenging or angry behaviors as long as they do not escalate into abusiveness or physical aggression. Instead, the therapist must work hard to control his own countertransferential anger or occasional sense of injustice and consistently convey acceptance of the client's affective responses. Such acceptance does not preclude gentle confrontation and clarification of angry expressions that actually mask fear or sadness, or more direct structuring responses to inappropriately threatening client responses.

Male Therapist, Female Client

Female survivor responses to male therapists are not as clearly delineated as those of male survivors regarding dominance of the therapeutic interaction. Specifically, as indicated in the previous section on female socialization, women who were sexually abused as children less frequently seek to be "one up" to male therapists, especially in terms of threatening, blustering, or aggressive behavior. However, their historically appropriate adversarial view of male–female interactions may be in force during therapy with male clinicians.

Some female abuse survivors seek to exert control over the psychotherapy session in the same ways that they may do in other interactions with powerful males, using sexual or stereotypical feminine behaviors to barter for acceptance, attention, and validation. This style of relating is different from that of the male survivor: While the male may attempt to dominate the session, the female survivor may view the interaction as having more to do with emotional survival. Stated differently, whereas the male survivor may try to fight to accomplish dominance, some female survivors are less interested in a battle than in avoiding male aggression—typically seeking to ingratiate or ally themselves with their assumed assailant as opposed to trying to vanquish him.

The preceding scenario is a generalization: There are women survivors who are aggressive (even violent) in sessions, clients who generally disdain males (although they are unlikely to seek therapy with a male in the first place), and a few who act in overtly sexual ways during treatment in a direct attempt to control and dominate the male therapist. There are also many women survivors for whom the male therapist's gender is of only minor importance. Nevertheless, the general trend seems to be for abuse trauma to heighten existing sex-role prescriptions regarding relations within and between the sexes, such that males are trained to convert dysphoria to aggression or dominance and females often learn to groom and maintain powerful males for safety and support.

The therapeutic implications of this role ownership for female survivors in treatment with male clinicians are significant. By virtue of his male stimulus value, the therapist may be blocked from making real therapeutic connections with the female survivor of male abuse. He is, in a sense, asking the female survivor to forget that he is a male, with all the power and dangerousness that she may associate with that gender. Thus, even the most nonexploitive, caring male begins treatment with female survivors of severe male abuse at a disadvantage: Until he proves otherwise (if he can), he may be seen as someone to service, maintain, or vilify rather than someone who can assist. Further, even his assistance may be relatively unhelpful if it reinforces the notion that mental health is a gift bestowed on a subordinate female by a powerful male with whom she is intimately connected.

The preceding analysis does not always hold. Many female sexual abuse survivors have been significantly helped by male therapists. It is important to note, however, that in many of these instances (a) the survivor was not extremely injured by her abuse (i.e., was healthy enough to see an exception to the rule of male dominance) and was not overly sexualized in her relationship to male authority; (b) the therapists in question were not predatory; and (c) abuse-gender issues were confronted, in some form, at various times during treatment.

As to the last point, there are several principles that should be attended to when male therapists see female abuse survivors (or, for that matter, nonabused women) in treatment. First and foremost, the clinician must be healthy enough, sexually and interpersonally, that he does not see female clients as potential objects for gratification of power, closeness, nurturance, or sexual needs. Thus, he should be clear regarding the boundaries between himself and his client, and should not exploit her in any manner, including for voyeuristic titillation or self-aggrandizement.

Second, he must be willing to assume that he is initially disabled by his gender stimulus value—that he must do extra work to arrive where competent female therapists begin (although female-female combinations have their own problems, as noted later in this chapter). The clinician who overlooks this point may miss the fact that his client may have been trained by victimization (and society) to placate and maintain males, often to her own detriment. As a result of this denial, he may subsequently be surprised by the transference and gender issues that "suddenly" arise.

Third, he must pay especially close attention to the client-therapist relationship, carefully reinforcing autonomy and self-affirming responses and gently discouraging, by nonparticipation, survivor behaviors that appear focused on the therapist's needs or well-being rather than her own.

Lastly, the therapist must be willing to take an unambiguous (albeit not always directly stated) stand against sexual aggression and implicit male social privilege relative to women. This last proviso is necessary because if this gender configuration is to work, the therapist must clearly demonstrate by his behavior that he does not subscribe to traditional masculine perspectives regarding the role and function of women. This position should not be used by the clinician to assert a holier-than-thou status relative to other men or stated in such a manner as to rule out client disagreement with the therapist's view of himself in this regard. Instead, the male therapist should pay particular attention to avoiding gender-based social and countertransferential responses to the survivor, such that his intention to provide nonsexist treatment is clearly apparent. In this way, the caring and noninvasive male therapist models the potential for more positive relationships with males in the future, as well as providing the opportunity to habituate and desensitize fearful responses to males in authority.

Female Therapist, Male Client

When the therapist is a woman and the survivor is a man, the dynamics that emerge are often a composite of those described earlier. On the one hand, the male client may seek to dominate the female therapist or respond to her as if she were a mother figure. Conversely, he may become seductive, seemingly interacting with the clinician solely in terms of her sexual stimulus value. In many instances, these patterns may be combined: The client may behave in a controlling, sexualized way, both flirting and challenging the therapist's status as "boss." Alternatively, he may combine the child role with elements of the dominant position: demanding maternal responses, and becoming angry and punitive if they are not forthcoming.

Male survivors (as well as other male clients) who respond to female therapists in a sexualizing or dominating manner are often using one of two related tactics. First, they may seek to reduce the threat posed by the woman clinician by accessing traditional rules regarding male–female relationships—hoping to negate her therapeutic power by placing her in the traditional role of sex object or subordinate. Typical statements by such clients are, "I'm sorry, I didn't hear what you said. I was distracted by your legs"; "Doctor, I think I'm falling in love with you. I can't get therapy from someone I feel this way about"; or "I can't believe you said that to me. Would your husband let you talk that way to him?"

The male survivor who responds in a sexualized or hypermasculine way also may be attempting to compensate for the fact that he was sexually victimized by a man. Expressing this history to a woman may prove embarrassing for some men who believe that their female therapist will see them as less masculine because of their victimization and the gender of their assailant. By responding to the clinician sexually or in a "macho" fashion, the client thus may communicate his desire to be seen as strong and virile rather than as a (by definition, less masculine) victim.

As opposed to the use of aggressive behavior to neutralize or impress the therapist, some male survivors, as noted earlier, respond to her as if she were an idealized mother. The client may regress during therapy, speak or act in a child-like fashion, or grow especially dependent and primitively demanding as treatment progresses. When this response is not primarily an "attachment transference," as described in chapter 5, motivation for this behavior pattern may be twofold. First, the choice to see the seemingly powerful clinician as a mother figure makes her safe and changes the agenda from one of working on one's issues to that of developing a source of much desired nurturance and comfort. Second, by converting the therapist to mother the male survivor reduces her power and credibility as a professional, given his typical view of mothering as a primitive, stereotypically feminine act.

There is another mother role beyond the idealized one, however. Male survivors who were sexually, physically, or emotionally abused by their mothers, or psychologically abandoned by them, are likely to view the female therapist as, at least to some extent, a perpetrator. In such instances, although there may (or may not) be sexualized or dominating client behavior, the client is likely to experience fear, anger, or abandonment issues. As a result, he may avoid the therapist, vilify her, have conditioned sexual responses to her, or may be especially preoccupied with her emotional and physical availability. These responses, which parallel some of those found in the male-therapist–female–client dynamic, require careful therapeutic attention to safety and boundary issues. The therapist should also be prepared for the possibility of sustained angry and punitive client behaviors—at least until the female therapist's nonabusive characteristics are more fully accepted by the client. These responses may easily fuel sexualized, aggressive, or controlling behaviors during treatment, as the male survivor—sometimes desperately—seeks ways to alter the power dynamic so that it is more in his favor and, therefore, "safer."

Thus, whether through sexualization, domination, or maternalization, some male survivors seek to decrease the threatening aspects of therapy by changing the role of the female therapist. Because (in addition to its irritating qualities for the clinician) this alteration is defensive—focusing the therapeutic process away from self-examination and emotional processing—it should be persistently discouraged. The message to be conveyed is that resolution of the male survivor's trauma will not be accomplished by exerting control over others or by strategically attenuating the impact of treatment. This message may be difficult for the client to apprehend completely, given the prodding of the male sex role to deal with anxiety through direct action or manipulation of the environment. The ultimate outcome may be positive, however, if the client can come to see his therapist not in the traditional guise of "woman" (sex object or mother) but rather as a respect-worthy guide to greater awareness and decreased pain.

Female Therapist, Female Client

Most writers on the treatment of sexual abuse effects suggest that this therapeutic pairing is the most advantageous (Blake-White & Kline, 1985; Herman, 1981) in the sense that female survivors are thought to be less defensive in therapy with women, and female therapists may be more empathic, aware of central women's issues, and least likely to victimize. Although this generalization fails in some specific instances, it has some overall validity based on male and female sex roles. When this pairing does encounter difficulties, it is often due to a set of potentially disruptive dynamics. Most frequently, these relate to ways in which the female therapist is seen as representing other, less positive women in the survivor's past and to sex-role prescriptions regarding female-female interactions.

As is also true for male survivors, women with abuse histories are prone to seeing female therapists as mother figures. The mother-child relationship appears to have more negative salience for female survivors, however, especially in terms of perceived abandonment and psychological abusiveness. Issues reflecting perceived maternal failure are well known to therapists who work with female incest survivors—although the father may have been the actual perpetrator, the mother is frequently most hated, often because she is seen as abandoning the survivor by not protecting her from abuse. As described earlier, this blaming of the mother for the father's behavior is sometimes technically unfair, although it may psychologically "true" for the survivor. This sense of having been abandoned, in turn, is often projected onto the female therapist, who may be simultaneously punished for her symbolic sins as well as tightly grasped to prevent what the survivor perceives as further betrayal.

Conflicts arising from the client's earlier psychological maltreatment by her mother are also common among female-female therapy dyads, even in those where sexual abuse was not present. The mother-daughter relationship is especially likely to be strained or adversarial, however, when sexual abuse is present in the home. As described in chapter 4, such families are often characterized by tension, conflict, hidden injuries, and skewed loyalties (Courtois, 1988; Harter, Alexander, & Neimeyer, 1988).

Although the mother is frequently unaware that her daughter is being sexually victimized by her husband or boyfriend, she may sense that some unusual connection between the two exists. Especially in cases in which the abuser is maltreating the mother as well, this "special" relationship may produce maternal jealousy, and the child may be punished or treated in an adversarial manner. Additionally, the mother may be psychologically abusive to the child independent of her partner's treatment of her. In either case, such maltreatment typically consists of rigid and contradictory rules regarding acceptable behavior, frequent criticisms and insults, and little emotional support.

This maternal maltreatment often has substantial impacts on how the survivor perceives the female clinician. She may be especially sensitive to what she believes to be critical or rejecting comments by her therapist, and she may make erroneous assumptions about the clinician's lack of empathy or caring for her. These cognitions may fuel reactive and defensive behaviors by the client, who is afraid to be vulnerable and yet desperately needs nurturance. Examples of such client behaviors are extensive quizzing of the therapist regarding her credentials and treatment approach, overly negative or defensive reaction to constructive feedback, testing of the therapist's commitment to her through various forms of acting out, and what may appear to be an almost paranoid suspicion about the clinician's motives for various statements or behaviors.

Beyond the effects of maternal abuse or neglect on treatment may be the client's stereotypic perception of the female clinician as either a competitor or, paradoxically, as irrelevant. Regarding the former, the adversarial focus of some abuse survivors cause them to see all women as competition for male attention. Thus, for example, the client may verbally or nonverbally compare her own attractiveness or stereotypic femininity to that of her therapist, the results of which may influence her subsequent interactions with the clinician during therapy.

If the therapist is perceived as more attractive to men, some heterosexual female clients may exhibit jealousy or bitterness and may assume that psychotherapy is unlikely to be successful. On a milder level, the client may make numerous comments, such as: "How would someone like you know how I feel"; or "If I had your body, I wouldn't be desperate either." If the client views herself as more physically attractive, she may subtly (or otherwise) use this "advantage" to nullify what she sees as her therapist's greater power. For example, she may discount clinician concerns about her compulsive sexuality, attraction to dominating males, or extreme male-focused orientation by implying that, being less attractive to men, the therapist is merely jealous about the client's greater status in a stereotypically feminine hierarchy. Similar comparisons may be made about the client's versus the therapist's relationship status, with the assumption that the possession of a man is a sign of success.

Finally, the survivor's sometimes extreme male orientation may cause her to devalue female therapists totally on the basis of their gender. Such clients may express disappointment that they "got stuck with a woman" as a therapist because they believe that women are less important, powerful, or valuable than men, and thus are less likely to be effective or interesting in therapy. This dynamic, incidentally, may create conflicts for those who assign clients to therapists (e.g., in clinics or counseling centers), for the client's insistence on a male therapist is sometimes evidence of her potentially greater need for a female one.

The various issues that arise in some female–female therapy dyads are thus primarily based on the survivor's familial, social, and abuse-related training regarding to other women. The female clinician must, therefore, view client reactions in these areas as potentially transferential and as information on fruitful areas for therapeutic attention. Such behaviors should additionally indicate to the therapist the importance of frequent clarification and support in work with such individuals. The therapist will typically work to alter her client's view of women and, therefore, of herself. Through her encounters with a strong and caring female role model who affirms the value of woman-ness, the survivor may slowly take back those parts of her identity that were distorted or negated by her victimization and traditional sex-role training.

SUMMARY

Although sexual abuse impacts on males and females in some of the same ways, the survivor's gender often affects how such abuse-related trauma will be experienced, expressed, and acted on. Further, it appears that if the survivor seeks out psychotherapy, sex-role stereotypes will additionally affect the course of treatment. These gender issues reflect the fact that sexual abuse occurs within a cultural context and highlight the importance of considering sex-role socialization, along with clinical issues, when working with sexual abuse survivors.

Therapist Issues 11

Working with sexual abuse survivors can be a gratifying experience for the psychotherapist. The opportunity to help someone grow through and past major psychological trauma can be a gift, one that bestows optimism and a sense of meaning to one's work. There is a "dark side" to such endeavors, however. The seemingly unending stream of anguished stories one listens to session after session, the personal impact of reliving other people's pain, and the frequent nonsupport of traditional mental health and social systems can easily have negative effects on the clinician and, therefore, potentially on his or her clients. Over time, the therapist may experience a growing sense of helplessness, anger, and disillusionment with the human condition. As noted by Summit (1987): "The usual anchors of training, authority, wisdom, and professional standards are elusive and contradictory for the sexual abuse specialist, and there is a compelling tendency to burn out, to abandon child advocacy, or to rely on the client for reassurance and reward" (p. 2). This final chapter is, therefore, written about the therapist. The most common pitfalls associated with this type of work are described, and several remedies are suggested.

ISOLATION

Whether employed within a mental health center, a psychiatric inpatient unit, or in private practice, the clinician working with sexual abuse survivors is prone to feelings of isolation. This is partially due to the nature of the work—it is difficult to share with others the actual experience of listening to client A as she describes her first violation at the hands of a formerly cherished father, or of client B who has been assaulted and abused by so many people that she seems to move through life as an object rather than a living person.

Psychotherapy with victims is a relatively autistic process, a closed system wherein the therapist unavoidably absorbs some portion of the client's pain and often is unable to unburden it to others fully. Many readers of this book, for example, are likely to have had the experience of discussing a particularly horrendous or saddening session with other therapists, only to find that their coworkers did not seem to have "enough" appreciation of the client's experience or of the therapist's reactions to it. Although some of this problem may reside in the ironically low level of supportiveness present in many mental health settings, there is also another process at work: Some of the experiences of those who treat survivors of violence just cannot be completely shared with anyone else. Not only is this truism salient with one's coworkers, it is also relevant to the therapist's home and social environment. As difficult as it may be to unburden oneself of "abuse stories" with other clinicians, it is almost impossible (and probably unfair, if not unethical) to do so with one's family, friends, or lover. The net result of this incommunicability is often a sense of working alone, without support.

Beyond the general sense of isolation experienced by anyone who listens to horrible stories on a regular basis, there is a separate process inherent in work with sexual abuse survivors: A society that discounts abuse and its effects will also tend to discount those who work with abuse victims. In consultation or supervision, the therapist's concerns about a given client may be dismissed by others, who may unduly pathologize the survivor, retreat to technical analyses, or use inappropriate or belittling humor. The clinician may find himself being paternalistically quizzed regarding the truthfulness of his client's statements, with the implication that he is overly credulous, and that the survivor's recollections are likely to be manipulations or false memories. It may be suggested that the clinician is being "hooked" or "pulled in" by the client by virtue of her apparent concern.

These subtle or overt disconfirmations of the clinician are frequently exacerbated when, as is often the case with survivors of severe abuse, the client makes a suicide attempt, acts out, or begins to make frequent telephone calls to the clinic. At such times, the tendency of some clinicians to see abuse reports as manipulations or attention-getting devices is reinforced, and it is often hinted to the therapist that she is "mismanaging the case" or "losing control of therapy." Such feedback, by nature of its implication that the therapist is not controlling the client well enough, is authoritarian and often antithetic to effective treatment of postabuse trauma. More generally, however, traditional responses to abuse survivors and those who would help them tends to drive the therapy underground: The clinician stops discussing upsetting cases with his or her peers and supervisors, and may strive to keep the client and therapy more or less a secret. Thus, the therapist finds herself cut off from standard resources, support, and professional consultation at a time when she needs them most.

IMPACT OF THE MATERIAL

In addition to the isolation felt by many therapists who work with abuse survivors, there is also the impact of the actual content of therapy. Therapeutic work with former sexual abuse victims routinely involves dealing with violence and cruelty at a level that many people would find incomprehensible. Repeated exposure to disclosures of violation, exploitation, and trauma can slowly produce a PTSD by proxy in the listener. It is not unusual, for example, for clinicians to report an increase in violent or distressing dreams as they work with abuse survivors or other victims of violence, nor is it uncommon for some therapists to become hypervigilant about personal danger in settings where they had previously felt unafraid (e.g., when alone at home, in empty streets, or even in previously safe-appearing relationships) (Pearlman & Saakvitne, 1995).

Ironically, it is likely that the clinician's therapeutic empathy makes him or her especially vulnerable to personally incorporating the trauma expressed by the client, thereby creating a secondary victim of the therapist. Signs of this process include increased irritability, free-floating anxiety, decreased ability to deal with stress appropriately, increased difficulties in personal relationships (including decreased sexual or romantic interest), and a general sense of being helpless to "fix" the pain and suffering around him or her. More basically, repeated contact with victims of violence often diminishes the therapist's belief in a just world, as was described earlier with reference to survivors. This may emerge as cynicism and chronic anger or helplessness regarding "the system," most combinations of which are detrimental to therapy and to the therapist.

As noted in chapter 5, because abuse-related material can slowly alter one's perspective regarding survivors, it is not uncommon to find workers in this area who are either overinvested or underinvested in their clients. Those who underinvest have, in most cases, dissociated from their client's trauma; similar to some abuse survivors, they become numb to what might otherwise invoke anxiety, anger, or depression. These clinicians may appear coolly professional or relatively disinterested in their client's history or pain. They may often come to see survivors as "cases," and respond to them in an unnecessarily detached or clinical manner. To create the maximal psychological distance from their clients' pain, such therapists may become invested in finding ways to view the abuse survivor as having caused or deserved her present predicament.

Their counterparts are those who overinvest, therapists who become extremely involved in their clients, often transcending the limits of appropriate therapist–client relationships. Such workers can frighten survivors with their intensity and personal involvement or may become highly parental and rescuing, to the highly inappropriate extent of taking clients home with them, lending them money, or seeing them in therapy many times a week. Their therapy style may become lecturing or advice giving, or they may become so uncritically supportive of their clients that they fail to confront or discuss inappropriate or destructive behavior. He or she may also unquestioningly accept all client disclosures as completely true, even if they contain contradictions or bizarre elements. In addition, such clinicians may express extreme anger at perpetrators, all parents, or all males, and may attempt to push their clients into equivalent affective states. Ultimately, they may come to believe that only they truly understand their clients and thus only they can treat them successfully.

This type of behavior, although understandable in light of the clinician's experience, is nevertheless nontherapeutic. It addresses the therapist's internal state rather than the survivor's current experience and often has the effect of infantilizing the client, or encouraging his or her dependence and regression. In extreme cases, the relationship ceases to be therapeutic and, instead, becomes intensely personal. At this point, the therapist has violated boundaries and misused the survivor's vulnerability in much the same way as did her childhood perpetrator.

IMPACT OF SOCIETAL RESPONSE

In the current zeitgeist, where therapists are increasingly subject to vitriolic attack by accused parents, the media, and nonclinical academics, the pressure on abuse-focused therapists sometimes seems unbearable. Most individuals who became therapists did so out of a desire to help people. When it became clear that such helping was associated with the isolation and stress described in the previous section, some clinicians eventually stopped working with survivors, or even left the profession. For those who remained, however, there was often an increased sense of doing the right thing, of persevering despite adversity, of banding together in a noble undertaking.

As certain elements of society have formed a more organized and coherent opposition to abuse work, however, the compound effects of work-related stress and social vilification have led to further difficulties for clinicians. Accused of implanting (rather than treating) abuse memories, of destroying innocent families, and threatened with lawsuits, therapists in the abuse area increasingly feel like villains rather than heroes. This perception of danger is no doubt increased by the parameters of the therapist's job description: Faced with daily evidence of the world's ability to be unfair, injurious, even perhaps evil, the clinician working with abuse victims is often easily led to believe that most people devalue or deride what he or she does professionally.

This alienation from society is increased by the fact that, as outlined in this book, a minority of therapists have, in fact, engaged in clinically inappropriate interventions. As a result, part of the social assault may feel indirectly deserved. At the same time, because most abuse therapists have not engaged in incompetent or malicious behavior, this attack on their credibility can feel especially unjust. Regardless of the clinician's feelings, however, the work must go on: One's clients must be seen, and, inevitably, further trauma must be addressed. The clinician is, therefore, forced to exhibit grace under fire, to continue to try to help, to be creative and available, all the while with a growing sense of concern and even fear for his or her own well-being, and for those he or she might someday be prevented from serving.

EFFECTS ON THE THERAPIST–REVISITED

As outlined earlier, it is clear that psychotherapy with abuse survivors is a double-edged sword for the clinician. On the one hand, the work is of great value and the benefits to the client are potentially immense. Conversely, such treatment is typically slow going, and the impacts on the therapist can be significant. Because it directly taps basic human concerns about responsibility, truth, safety versus danger, and love versus betrayal, child abuse can evoke adverse reactions in many clinicians—responses that can easily interfere with treatment.

As described in this chapter, the work itself is often traumatizing, especially when one's case load consists primarily of survivors. Clinician empathy, as noted earlier, may support the therapist's internalization of the former victim's injury. In addition, the prevalence of child victimization in our society—whether it be sexual molestation, physical maltreatment, or emotional abuse—usually means that the therapist herself has points of psychic vulnerability based on painful childhood experience. Thus, client trauma may open up old wounds in the clinician, and potentially cause him or her to lose perspective.

Finally, our culture impacts on therapists, just as it does victims and abusers. The clinician's membership in society—yet his or her investment in combating some of its injustices—can result in a tremendous sense of abandonment when, understandably, elements of society defend themselves by attacking him or her. The abuse-focused clinician is, in some strange sense, attempting to confront society with its sins while, at the same time, seeking acceptance from it.

A result of these various forces and contradictions is stress on the therapist as she or he tries to maintain objectivity during the psychotherapy process. To the extent that he or she is successful, the client may grow and recover, whereas the undersupported therapist may become increasingly drained and "burned out." Conversely, if the therapist is unsuccessful in maintaining clinical objectivity, both client and clinician will suffer.

The following section offers the possibility of a third option: activities and interventions that help to center and support the therapist, thereby permitting him to assist others while she herself grows stronger.

Remedies

One's Own Therapy

It is probably a good idea for any mental health worker to have undergone psychotherapy as a client. Not only does therapy reveal to the clinician what being a client feels like, it also helps him to understand and control what might otherwise be nontherapeutic responses to his client's disclosures and behaviors. As helpful as therapy may be for the general clinician, it becomes even more important for those who work with abuse survivors. Specifically, as noted earlier, one's unresolved childhood experiences are likely to stimulate countertransferential reactions to abuse-related client material. Psychotherapy, by virtue of its emphasis on self-awareness and the processing of personal history, can help the clinician to see her client more clearly and to respond less defensively to client behavior during treatment.

Among the issues that the therapist in therapy might consider addressing in this regard are (a) the tendency to impose his own childhood-based perceptions (such as helplessness or authority issues) onto his client; (b) his potential for defensive responding to client anger and criticism, as if the client has suddenly become a childhood abuser; (c) his need to control restimulated anxiety during therapy by keeping the client from addressing the full extent of her or his victimization; and (d) his own socially learned identification with the aggressor that might lead him to support the actions of his client's perpetrator. More generally, the task for the therapist-as-client is to come to terms with her childhood history, such that she no longer projects early injuries onto others—most notably her clients.

In addition to one's own history, therapists whose psychotherapy also examines gender issues may have the opportunity to confront the effects of traditional sex-role socialization on their behavior as clinicians. For males, this may involve the development of greater empathy for women and children, the opportunity to learn how to relate intimately to others without the intrusion of sexual issues, and the chance to examine how he too has been socialized to victimize others (e.g., via sexual coercion, excessive competition, or dominance over those with lesser social power, such as one's wife or children). Female therapists, conversely, may learn to confront socially trained passivity and related assumptions regarding the appropriateness of male dominance, and may discover the cognitive shift required to identify with her female client's strengths rather than with her fears or helplessness.

Finally, his or her own psychotherapy can provide the therapist with an ongoing sounding board during work with survivors. Unlike supervision alone, such therapy allows the therapist as client to explore in depth his reactions to the clients' victimization histories, and to do so in light of his own personal history and issues. This process offers the therapist an opportunity to remain centered and focused during particularly impactful or personally confusing sessions with her client. A beneficial side effect of this process is that such sessions may serve as a source of stimuli for the clinician's own therapy by restimulating avoided childhood memories and by the sustained attention to abuse-related concerns that working with survivors demands.

Sharing the Load

Beyond one's own psychotherapy, the difficulties involved in working with survivors can be lessened by regular consultation with other abuse-focused clinicians. Unlike interactions with those who question the validity of abuse and its effects, debriefing a particularly intense session with a like-minded therapist can decrease considerably the sense of isolation and responsibility associated with this work. As clinicians in this area will attest, an important part of this process seems to be, within the limits of confidentiality, the sharing of "horror stories" with one another. To the outsider, such interactions might seem likely to intensify the worker's stress because one might assume that each therapist would incorporate the other's worst experiences. Instead, this activity frequently produces a paradoxical calming effect and often serves to restore perspective. The clinician typically rediscovers that she is not alone in this task, that others are grappling with equally disturbing scenarios, and that this sort of work is surmountable and survivable. Graphic descriptions of one's client's victimization undoubtedly also serves as a form of catharsis and emotional processing, as the clinician works to desensitize and integrate painful material. In this way, what otherwise might appear to be group self-flagellation or trauma overload operates as a way of accommodating to repeated horror stories, and serves to reassure the clinician that "I am not alone in this," "other people's clients are equally distressed," or even "I am not doing something wrong by being privy to such pain."

As useful as such group sharing is, therapists who work with survivors of violence should also consider regular, scheduled sessions with a consultant or clinical supervisor who is experienced with former abuse victims. Ideally occurring on a weekly basis for 1 to 1½ hours, the consultation session is an opportunity for the clinician to discuss upsetting, frustrating, or irritating interactions with clients regularly, to examine the impact of such work on his or her own psyche, and to hear useful suggestions and perspectives from the consultant regarding what is transpiring and what to do next. By virtue of their predictable regularity, these sessions come to be relied on by the therapist, who knows that within a few days or hours she will have someone to share with and, if need be, lean on and gain perspective.

It is difficult to emphasize enough the helpfulness of regularly scheduled consultation or supervision sessions for those who work with survivors of severe child maltreatment. In my opinion, this is one of the most important mechanisms that an agency, clinic, or hospital administration can offer its therapists if they wish to decrease the rate of burnout and increase the quality of service. Similarly, I suggest that those in private practice consider hiring a clinical consultant who will meet with them on a regular basis, in the same way that they might hire a receptionist or accountant. Although such consultation is not imperative for all practices, it is almost always helpful.

Beyond the salutary effects of debriefing and consultation, networking with clinicians in other settings and locations can also be helpful. This may be accomplished by having monthly or bimonthly meetings with abuse therapists from other local centers or practices, during which time mechanisms for transfer of clients, interagency disputes, and common endeavors can be discussed. Such settings also have the positive effect of decreasing the insularity of a given treatment center or office; by listening to the similar concerns and experiences of workers in other agencies or clinics, clinicians from a given location are less likely to feel as if they are the only experts on survivor treatment in the city and may be less prone to adopt a siege mentality regarding contact with other helpers.

On a broader scale, networking should include attendance at state, provincial, or national conventions on child abuse and psychological trauma. Attendance at such meetings often engenders a feeling of being part of a movement to help children and survivors, and almost inevitably solidifies one's sense of identity as a specialist in an important area. Additionally, this form of networking allows the clinician to see the "big picture" regarding the amelioration of child maltreatment and its effects, a process that often lessens the perceived seriousness of individual disappointments or political bickering back home. Finally, membership in larger organizations may decrease the sense of isolation, rejection, and fearfulness associated with criticism by the media and accused parent advocacy groups.

Mixed Case Loads

No matter how much one chooses to specialize in the treatment of abuse effects, those clinicians who have a choice regarding their caseloads should avoid seeing solely victims of violence—let alone solely sexual abuse survivors. Continual and exclusive work with people who have been intentionally injured or exploited by others can easily alter one's perceptions, in and out of therapy. As described earlier in this chapter, such exclusivity may result in views of the world as inherently dangerous, relationships as usually adversarial, and the future as often bleak.

These distortions in perception, along with the emotional impact of continual exposure to severely injured clients, can combine to produce therapists who are especially pessimistic and, in some sense, "shell-shocked" by their profession. For this reason, most successful (i.e., helpful and healthy) clinicians include some relatively high functioning, less abused clients in their caseload. Such clients are often more free to be creative and engaging than survivors of extreme abuse, and usually are far less demanding of the therapist's time and energy. Work with these people ideally reminds the therapist that, among other things, some parents are not harmful to their children, growth is as important as recovery, and psychotherapy can be a more immediately helpful endeavor.

Social Partitions

As is also true for some other professions (e.g., police and ER personnel), mental health clinicians tend to interact socially with other clinicians. Given the social isolation often associated with being an abuse-focused therapist, workers in this area may especially limit their contacts to others who treat abuse survivors, and devote much of their time to thinking and talking about interpersonal violence and, perhaps, societal backlash against their work with survivors. The positive aspects of restricting one's social circle include not having to defend one's work to others, having friends and partners who understand what one is going through with difficult clients, and the general warm feeling that accompanies relationships in a close-knit, movement-oriented community. Unfortunately, as reinforcing as such connections may be, chronic preoccupation with abuse-related issues and abuse-focused coworkers can have negative consequences, much in the same way as occurs when one's caseload is restricted to survivors.

Perhaps the most important of these effects is on the therapist's world view. By relating more or less exclusively to other abuse-specialized psychotherapists and spending much of one's time discussing abuse-related issues, the susceptible clinician may easily come to believe that everyone is either a victim, perpetrator, therapist, or critic, or some combination of all four. A major impact of this assumption is the tendency to see violence, adversariality, or tragedy in all things, and thereby miss the many opportunities to love, laugh, be silly, and appreciate beauty around him or her.

This process, which can reverberate and amplify within an abuse-focused social group, may interfere with the therapist's ability to regenerate his or her excitement about life, and may foster cynicism or helplessness. Ultimately, by virtue of the power of abuse-related issues and the therapist's reflexive tendency to remain with others who share her commitment, some clinicians extend the emotional impact of their work to most of their waking hours. When this occurs, the therapist is even more prone to the problems outlined in this chapter.

The solution to overinvestment in abuse issues is not to blame oneself for caring so deeply, nor is it to abandon the field. Instead, the clinician is advised to partition her or his life: focusing on victimization during one's work and living a "regular" life outside of it. Thus, although consultation, debriefing, and networking are antidotal to burnout during work, different approaches are indicated when one is not working. There are at least three remedies that appear to be especially useful in this regard: (a) reducing abuse-related discussions and activities during social and nonworking hours, (b) becoming involved in noncognitive and physically demanding activities, and (c) taking "mental health breaks."

The first suggestion implies a different approach to socializing with friends. The therapist is counseled to widen her or his social circle—intentionally seeking out friendships with artists, architects, trade or business people, and others who live lives substantially different from one's own. Similarly, social activities with other therapists should explicitly avoid extended shop-talk sessions and, instead, be approached as opportunities to relax, enjoy one another, expand one's horizons, and (dare it be said in such a serious world) have fun.

The second recommendation reflects the notion that psychotherapy is primarily a cognitive task, involving words, thoughts, and ideas as vehicles for emotional growth. Because of this, some psychotherapists become overdeveloped cognitively: tending to want to analyze and intellectually understand (if not control) much of what they encounter. This predisposition to thinking and talking rather than acting or feeling can dominate one's daily life and may cause the clinician to forget that he or she is a living organism who has inherent needs for physical exercise and, possibly, adventure. When unmet, these needs may produce chronic dysphoria—a process that is antithetic to recovery from the stress of treating abuse trauma.

For this reason, the clinician may choose to engage in physically demanding activities on a regular basis, such as daily walks, running, hiking, or basketball. Many therapists have noted that aerobic activities are effective "thought interrupters" and tension reducers, allowing the clinician to finally stop ruminating over—and reacting to—the worst sessions or stories of the day. Regular exercise has been shown to decrease stress levels and to inhibit subsequent overreaction to stressful events as well.

The last suggestion involves "mental health breaks." This term refers to intentional interruptions of one's occupational routine to allow recovery from work-related stress. As this concept relates to abuse therapists, it is recommended that psychotherapists take relatively frequent (e.g., bimonthly) "minivacations" of several days, preferably out of town, during which time little or no attention is paid to therapy or abuse. Although this regimen might appear extravagant to clinic administrators, my previous experience as an agency clinical director taught me that burnout, excessive sick days, and excessive staff conflict could sometimes be reduced by proactively intervening in work-related stress. For example, a therapist who takes a "three-day weekend" every several months may be considerably less likely to require more days in sick leave and may be more able to work efficiently with abuse survivors in the time that he or she does spend in the clinic.

Macrointerventions

The final remedy presented in this chapter may be less intuitively obvious than those described thus far. It approaches the stressfulness of work with abuse survivors not just by lessening the load or by providing more resources but also by increasing the meaningfulness of the intervention process. Specifically, one of the major stressors involved in helping victims of violence is the fact that such work is primarily reactive—we strive to help those who have been hurt, all the while knowing that many more are being victimized even as we do so. As a well-known community psychologist once said, psychotherapy is like pulling drowning people out of a river, never having the time to go upstream and stop whomever is pushing them in. Knowing that she can never catch up with the victim-producing process, the clinician is left with helping those who have already been injured. This awareness can be demoralizing, and can easily lead to feelings of inadequacy and helplessness.

Thus, the last recommendation to be offered here is to travel upriver. Rather than concentrating all of his or her efforts on treating abuse trauma, the clinician may experience some real satisfaction in broader (macro) prevention efforts as well. Because the sexual victimization of children is, to some extent, the result of a violent culture, such efforts may involve a variety of social interventions, ranging from public education or working with action groups for legislative change to involvement in antisexism school curriculum. Additionally, the therapist may choose to present workshops on the effects and treatment of child abuse, or write papers or books on sexual victimization for mental health workers. Whatever the activity, the sense that one is directly addressing the problem—rather than solely treating its effects—can be a powerful antidote to feelings of helplessness.

SUMMARY

This chapter has been about the process of helping sexual abuse survivors as it impacts on the therapist. It is suggested that the clinician, as a human being, both brings her own issues into treatment and is affected by the pain she confronts during that process, whether it be the horrific nature of a specific client disclosure or an especially unfair attack by the media. As a person, as opposed to a mere therapeutic instrument, the therapist must understand his strengths and limitations, and should not deceive himself that psychotherapy is anything but a subjective, highly personal process. Because of this, it is the psychotherapist's responsibility to her client—and to herself—to remain psychologically healthy, and to be relatively aware of her own concerns, defenses, and behaviors as they interact with the client's. If this can be accomplished, such treatment will benefit not only the client but the therapist as well.

Appendix

Assessing the Long-term Effects of
Sexual Abuse with
The Trauma Symptom Inventory (TSI)

Diana Elliott and John Briere

This appendix presents information on a standardized psychological test of psychological trauma that may be especially useful in assessing the long-term impacts of sexual abuse. The TSI (Briere, 1995) is the result of a multiyear project to expand and improve the Trauma Symptom Checklist (TSC-33/40; Briere & Runtz, 1989; Elliott & Briere, 1992), a research instrument presented in the appendix of the last edition of this book.

Although the TSI is not the only measure of posttraumatic or victimization-related difficulties (Foa, Riggs, Dancu, & Rothbaum, 1993; Foy, Sipprelle, Rueger, & Carroll, 1984; Horowitz, Wilner, & Alvarez, 1979), its multiscale nature, positive psychometrics, and standardization allows for specific evaluation of the wide range of affective, posttraumatic, sexual, behavioral, and self-related symptoms associated with severe childhood sexual abuse in adults. Psychologists and others qualified to provide psychological assessment may find that the TSI, especially in conjunction with the MMPI-2, MCMI-III, PAI (Personality Assessment Inventory, Morey 1991), or Rorschach, provides detailed and helpful psychometric information on postabuse functioning not easily obtained otherwise (Briere, 1995, in press, a).

This Appendix describes the TSI, outlines its psychometric characteristics, and provides information on the average response of sexually abused and nonabused individuals in clinical samples. The

217

interested reader is referred to Briere (1995) and Briere, Elliott, Harris, and Cotman (1995) for further information on the TSI and its performance regarding interpersonal trauma.

DESCRIPTION OF THE TRAUMA
SYMPTOM INVENTORY

The TSI is a 100-item test of posttraumatic stress and other psychological sequelae of traumatic events, available in hand-scorable and computer-scored versions. It is intended for use in the evaluation of acute and chronic traumatic symptomatology, including the lasting sequelae of childhood abuse and other early traumatic events, as well as the more acute effects of rape, spouse abuse, physical assault, major accidents, and natural disasters.

The items of the TSI are contained in a reusable test booklet, available from Psychological Assessment Resources.[*] Each symptom item is rated according to how often it has occurred over the prior 6 months, using a 4-point scale ranging from 0 ("never") to 3 ("often").

The TSI has been standardized on a representative sample of 836 men and women from the general population, age 18 or older, and includes separate military norms based on data from 3,659 male and female Navy recruits. Separate norms are provided for different combinations of sex and age (males and females under 55 years vs. 55 years and older), and race-related variations are considered.

The TSI has three validity scales and ten clinical scales[**], as presented below in Table A.1.

Psychometric characteristics
of the Trauma Symptom Inventory

The clinical scales of the TSI are internally consistent (mean αs of .86, .87, .84, and .84 in general population, clinical, university, and

---

[*]P.O. Box 998, Odessa, FL 33556-9901.
[**]The computer-scored version (Briere & P.A.R. staff, 1995) (Psychological Assessment Resources) generates three additional summary scales (Truama, Self, and Dysphoria) above and beyond the 10 clinical scales available in the hand-scored version.

military samples, respectively), and exhibit convergent, predictive, and incremental validity (Briere, 1995b). The validity scales demonstrate reasonable convergence with similar scales in other measures.

TSI T-scores are calculated so as to have a mean of 50 and a standard deviation of 10, and provide information about the individual's scores on each scale relative to those in the general population. T-scores at or above 65 are considered clinically elevated on the TSI. The interested reader is referred to the *TSI Professional Manual* for demographic and standardization information on the normative samples, as well as more detailed information on the TSI as it relates to various traumatized groups.

Association With Sexual Abuse Trauma in a Clinical Sample

Because this book specifically addresses the long-term effects of sexual abuse in psychotherapy clients, Tables A.2 and A.3 present previously unpublished TSI T-score data for sexually abused and nonabused subjects in 391 clinical subjects (see Briere et al., [1995] for further details on this sample).

Sixty-seven percent of these subjects were recruited by therapists from their outpatient clinical practices (203 females and 44 males), and 33% were from two general psychiatric inpatient units (101 females and 43 males). The mean age of subjects in the combined clinical sample was 36 years ($SD = 9.5$; range = 18 to 54). Of the total sample, 316 (81%) were White, 44 (11%) were Hispanic, 26 (7%) were African American/Black, and 5 (1%) were Asian. Subjects were identified as former sexual abuse victims if they reported actual sexual contact before age 17 that was physically forced or that occurred with someone 5 or more years older. A history of childhood sexual abuse was reported by 69% of the women ($n = 211$) and 28% of the men ($n = 24$).

Multivariate and univariate analyses of variance indicate that females scored higher than males on two scales, AA and DIS ($F[10,374] = 3.04$, $p < .001$), inpatients scored higher than outpatients on all scales ($F [10,374] = 7.27$, $p < .001$), and sexual abuse survivors scored higher on all scales than did those without a sexual abuse history ($F [10,374] = 6.70$, $p < .001$). There were no interactions between these variables. Female inpatient sexual abuse survivors scored in the clinical range

Table A.1 Trauma Symptom Inventory scales

Scale type	Scale	Symptom or response measured
Validity	Response Level (RL)	A tendency toward defensiveness, a general underendorsement response set, or a need to appear unusually symptom free
	Atypical Response (ATR)	A tendency to report unusual experiences, often associated with psychosis or extreme distress, a general overendorsement response set, or an attempt to appear especially disturbed or dysfunctional
	Inconsistent Response (INC)	A tendency to respond in an inconsistent or contradictory manner to Trauma Symptom Inventory TSI items, potentially reflecting random item endorsement, attention or concentration problems, or reading/language difficulties
Clinical	Anxious Arousal (AA)	Symptoms of anxiety, especially those associated with posttraumatic hyperarousal (e.g., jumpiness and tension)
	Depression (D)	Depressive symptomatology, both in terms of mood state (e.g., sadness) and depressive cognitive distortions (e.g., hopelessness)
	Anger/Irritability (AI)	Self-reported angry or irritable affect, as well as associated angry cognitions and behavior
	Intrusive Experiences (IE)	Intrusive symptoms associated with posttraumatic stress, such as flashbacks, nightmares, and intrusive thoughts

Defensive Avoidance (DA)	Posttraumatic avoidance, both cognitive (e.g., pushing painful thoughts or memories out of one's mind) and behavioral (e.g., avoidance of stimuli reminiscent of a traumatic event)
Dissociation (DIS)	Dissociative symptomatology, such as depersonalization, derealization, out-of-body experiences, and psychic numbing
Sexual Concerns (SC)	Self-reported sexual distress, such as sexual dissatisfaction, sexual dysfunction, and unwanted sexual thoughts or feelings
Dysfunctional Sexual Behavior (DSB)	Sexual behavior that is in some way dysfunctional, either because of its indiscriminate quality, its potential for self-harm, or its inappropriate use to accomplish nonsexual goals
Impaired Self-Reference (TRB)	Problems in the "self" domain, such as identity confusion, self-other disturbance, and a relative lack of self-support
Tension Reduction (TRB)	A tendency to turn to external methods of reducing internal tension or distress, such as self-mutilation, angry outbursts, "manipulative" behavior, and suicide threats

Table A.2 Mean Female TSI T-Scores According to
Sexual Abuse History and Inpatient vs. Outpatient Status (N = 304).

| | Outpatient females | | | | Inpatient females | | | |
| | No CSA (N = 55) | | CSA (N = 148) | | No CSA (N = 38) | | CSA (N = 63) | |
Scale	M	SD	M	SD	M	SD	M	SD
Anxious Arousal	56.0	(10.8)	62.5	(10.2)	61.2	(9.2)	66.8	(9.0)
Depression	53.3	(9.5)	61.6	(10.1)	64.8	(7.6)	70.0	(7.2)
Anger/Irritability	53.3	(9.0)	60.8	(10.0)	59.4	(10.8)	62.9	(9.7)
Intrusive Experiences	52.8	(10.5)	62.4	(11.1)	55.0	(10.4)	64.4	(11.8)
Defensive Avoidance	53.6	(9.2)	59.9	(9.9)	56.8	(10.1)	65.2	(7.8)
Dissociation	55.0	(10.5)	65.8	(12.8)	62.0	(10.6)	71.5	(11.5)
Sexual Concerns	53.6	(10.3)	63.8	(13.0)	54.7	(12.0)	65.0	(15.0)
Dysfunctional Sexual Behavior	50.1	(9.8)	56.1	(14.9)	52.7	(10.0)	59.7	(17.7)
Impaired Self-Reference	57.7	(10.3)	63.6	(10.5)	64.0	(8.8)	68.5	(9.3)
Tension-Reduction Behavior	52.2	(8.6)	60.6	(14.0)	59.3	(11.5)	67.7	(14.5)

Note. TSI = Trauma Symptom Inventory; CSA = Childhood Sexual Abuse; M = Mean; SD = Standard Deviation.

Table A.3 Mean Male TSI T-Scores According to Sexual Abuse History and Inpatient vs. Outpatient Status (N = 87).

Scale	Outpatient males				Inpatient males			
	No CSA (N = 29)		CSA (N = 15)		No CSA (N = 34)		CSA (N = 9)	
	M	SD	M	SD	M	SD	M	SD
Anxious Arousal	47.1	(4.4)	58.1	(10.9)	61.3	(11.3)	59.3	(10.5)
Depression	50.5	(7.3)	60.4	(12.2)	61.9	(12.6)	69.0	(7.6)
Anger/Irritability	53.8	(10.2)	58.7	(8.0)	60.1	(10.8)	62.1	(10.0)
Intrusive Experiences	46.5	(6.7)	57.6	(10.8)	57.2	(11.6)	64.3	(10.9)
Defensive Avoidance	48.3	(6.8)	61.9	(6.6)	59.2	(10.7)	63.8	(4.4)
Dissociation	49.8	(6.7)	60.4	(13.4)	61.3	(14.4)	61.2	(17.6)
Sexual Concerns	46.6	(5.2)	62.9	(14.4)	58.4	(15.1)	66.1	(12.6)
Dysfunctional Sexual Behavior	45.8	(3.1)	60.5	(17.5)	57.9	(14.1)	61.4	(15.1)
Impaired Self-Reference	52.8	(8.1)	65.4	(14.6)	62.9	(11.4)	65.2	(13.1)
Tension-Reduction Behavior	50.3	(7.9)	61.8	(8.6)	60.6	(11.3)	67.1	(18.7)

Note. TSI = Trauma Symptom Inventory; CSA = Childhood Sexual Abuse; M = Mean; SD = Standard Deviation.

($T > 64$) on seven TSI scales: Anxious Arousal, Depression, Defensive Avoidance, Dissociation, Sexual Concerns, Impaired Self-Reference, and Tension-Reduction Behavior. Male inpatient sexual abuse survivors scored in the clinical range on three scales: Depression, Impaired Self-Reference, and Tension-Reduction Behavior.

These data suggest that sexual abuse survivors score considerably higher on the TSI than do those without a sexual abuse history. Nonabused individuals, whether in outpatient or inpatient samples, had no TSI scale scores in the clinical range, whereas sexually abused individuals (especially in the inpatient samples) had several clinical elevations. These findings are all the more significant because all subjects (including the comparison group) in this study were from clinical settings, and thus were more likely—as a group—to have symptoms relative to nonclinical groups.

The data presented thus far refers to average scores on the TSI as a function of sexual abuse history. It is at the individual level, however, that the clinician uses TSI results, often to graph a multiscale symptom profile. Presented below is a typical profile for a survivor of severe childhood sexual abuse, adapted from the *TSI Professional Manual* (Briere, 1995b).

> Ms. K., a subject in the TSI clinical trials, is a 46-year-old, White, single woman who seeks psychotherapy for self-destructive impulses and relationship problems. She reports a long childhood history of incestuous abuse by her father but no major adult traumas. On the MMPI-2, this woman had a 2-7-8 profile and no significant elevations on either MMPI PTSD scale. Figure A.1 presents her TSI profile.
>
> This is a valid profile, although ATR and INC are slightly above normal. Ms. K. has six scales in the clinical range (ISR, DIS, TRB, DSB, SC, and D; see Table A. for abbreviations). She endorses critical items involving getting into trouble because of sex and involvement in self-mutilatory behavior. This profile suggests that Ms. K. has significant symptomatology in the area of identity and self-awareness, tends to use tension-reduction behaviors to deal with internal distress (e.g., through sex and self-mutilation), and has numerous sexual concerns and difficulties. She also reports considerable dissociative symptomatology, as well as a moderate level of depression. The DIS-DSB-SC component of this profile is often associated with excessive or maladaptive sexual behavior that may be seen by the individual as both shameful

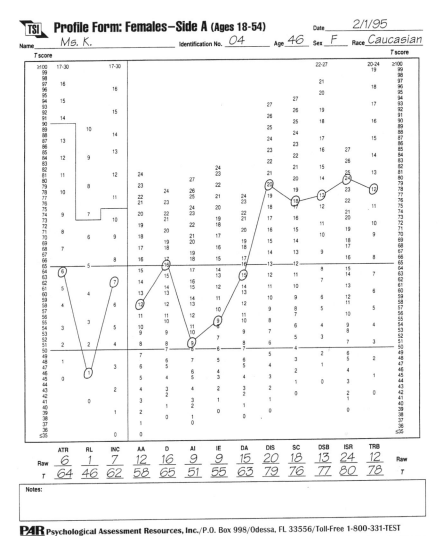

Figure A.1 Trauma Symptom Inventory for 46-year-old, White, single woman. *From Trauma Symptom Inventory Professional Manual. Copyright © 1995 by Psychological Assessment Resources, Inc. Reprinted with permission of the publisher.*

and uncontrollable. As suggested by chapters 1 to 3, this constellation of symptoms and behaviors is not uncommon among those who have experienced chronic and severe childhood sexual abuse.

The clinical implications of this profile are several. Ms. K. appears to be in considerable distress, primarily in the areas of self-functioning and sexuality. She may have received a diagnosis of borderline personality disorder or traits, and is likely to be seen by her therapist as prone to self-destructive and self-defeating behavior. Acting out (tension reduction) under stress is probably a common occurrence for Ms. K., and thus she should be approached with special attention to the therapeutic window dynamics described in earlier chapters (e.g., intensity control, and attention to the balance between self-resources and traumatic distress). Her report of self-mutilatory behavior, albeit common in survivors of prolonged sexual abuse, is further indicative of her need for relatively primitive tension reduction. Such ongoing self-injury should be monitored for its severity, disfigurement potential, potential lethality, and implicit suggestion of overwhelming internal distress. Her sexual concerns and behaviors indicate major difficulties in this area, including the possibility of involvement in unsafe sexual practices. Because Ms. K. has elevations on both depression and tension reduction, suicidality is also a possibility and should be monitored regularly. Fortunately, she endorsed no critical items concerned with suicidality or wanting to die.

Individuals similar to Ms. K. usually require considerable time in therapy, not only because of the severity of their difficulties but also as a result of their regular involvement in avoidance behavior (e.g., dissociation and tension reduction): activities that might easily interfere with treatment. Effective therapy would ideally focus first on the development of self-care strategies, increased affect regulation skills, and more positive coping responses, after which the posttraumatic components of her symptomatology could be carefully processed and desensitized. Although her self-difficulties suggest an extended course of treatment, her ultimate prognosis might well be positive. Critical in this regard would be Ms. K.'s ability to tolerate the anxiety and restimulated distress associated with a sustained therapeutic relationship, and the clinician's willingness to move slowly and carefully, providing the opportunity for growth and resolution in the context of continuing safety.

References

Abbott, B. R. (1995). Group therapy. In C. Classen (Ed.). *Treating women molested in childhood.* San Francisco: Jossey-Bass.

Abney, V. A., Yang, J. A., & Paulson, M. J. (1992). Transference and countertransference issues unique to long-term group psychotherapy of adult women molested as children: Trials and rewards. *Journal of Interpersonal Violence, 7,* 559–569.

Abueg, F. R., & Fairbank, J. A. (1992). Behavioral treatment of posttraumatic stress disorder and co-occurring substance abuse. In P.A. Saigh (Ed.), *Posttraumatic stress disorder: A behavioral approach to assessment and treatment* (pp. 111–146). Needham Heights, MA: Allyn & Bacon.

Alexander, P.C. (1992). Effect of incest on self and social functioning: A developmental psychopathology perspective. *Journal of Consulting and Clinical Psychology, 60,* 185–219

Alpert, J. L., & Paulson, A. (1990). Graduate-level education and training in child sexual abuse. *Professional Psychology: Research and Practice, 21,* 366–371.

American Psychiatric Association. (1994). *Diagnostic and statistical manual of mental disorders (4th ed.).* Washington, DC: Author.

Anderson, G., Yasenik, L., & Ross, C. (1993). Dissociative experiences and disorders among women who identify themselves as sexual abuse survivors. *Child Abuse & Neglect, 17,* 677–686.

Armstrong, L. (1983). *The home front.* New York: McGraw-Hill.

Astin, M. C., Layne, C. M., Camilleri, A. J., & Foy, D. W. (1994). Posttraumatic stress disorder in victimization-related traumata. In J. Briere

(Ed.), *Violent victimization: Assessment and treatment.* San Francisco: Jossey-Bass.

Bagley, C. (1984). Mental health and the in-family sexual abuse of children and adolescents. *Canada's Mental Health, June,* 17–23.

Bagley, C. (1991). The prevalence and mental health sequels of child sexual abuse in a community sample of women aged 18 to 27. *Canadian Journal of Community Mental Health, 10,* 103–116.

Bagley, C., & Ramsay, R. (1986). Disrupted childhood and vulnerability to sexual assault: Long-term sequels with implications for counselling. *Social Work and Human Sexuality, 4,* 33–48.

Bagley, C., & Young, L. (1987). Juvenile prostitution and child sexual abuse: A controlled study. *Canadian Journal of Community Mental Health, 6,* 5–26.

Beck, A. T. (1967). *Depression: Clinical, experimental and theoretical aspects.* New York: Harper & Row.

Beck, A. T., Emory, G., & Greenberg, R. L. (1985). *Anxiety disorders and phobias: A cognitive perspective.* New York: Basic Books.

Becker, J., Skinner, L., Abel, G., & Treacy, E. (1982). Incidence and types of sexual dysfunctions in rape and incest victims. *Journal of Sex and Marital Therapy, 8,* 65–74.

Bem, S. L., & Lenney, E. (1976). Sex typing and the avoidance of cross-sex behavior. *Journal of Personality and Social Psychology, 33,* 48–54.

Berliner, L., (in press). Trauma specific therapy for sexually abused children. In D. Wolfe & R. McMahon (Eds.), *Proceedings of the 27th Banff International Conference on Behavioral Science.*

Berliner, L., & Elliott, D. M. (1996). Sexual abuse of children. In J. Briere, L. Berliner, J. Bulkley, C. Jenny, & T. Reid (Eds.), *The APSAC handbook on child maltreatment.* Newbury Park, CA: Sage.

Berliner, L., & Wheeler, J. R. (1987). Treating the effects of sexual abuse on children. *Journal of Interpersonal Violence, 2,* 415–434.

Blake-White, J., & Kline, C. M. (1985). Treating the dissociative process in adult victims of childhood incest. *Social Casework: The Journal of Contemporary Social Work, 66,* 394–402.

Blatt, S. J., Wein, S. J., Chevron, E., & Quinlan, D. M. (1979). Parental representations and depression in normal young adults. *Journal of Abnormal Psychology, 88,* 388–397.

Bograd, M. (1984). Family systems approach to wife battering: A feminist critique. *American Journal of Orthopsychiatry, 54,* 558–568.

Bowen, G. R., & Lambert, J. A. (1986). Systematic desensitization therapy with post-traumatic stress disorder cases. In C. R. Figley (Ed.), *Trauma and its wake* (Vol. 2). New York: Brunner/Mazel.

Bowlby, J. (1973). *Attachment and loss: Vol. 2. Separation: Anxiety and anger.* London: Hogarth.

Bowlby, J. (1988). *A secure base: Parent-child attachment and healthy human development.* New York: Basic Books.

Briere, J. (1987). Predicting likelihood of battering: Attitudes and childhood experiences. *Journal of Research in Personality, 21,* 61–69.

Briere, J. (1988). The long-term clinical correlates of childhood sexual victimization. *New York Academy of Sciences, 528,* 327–334.

Briere, J. (1992a). *Child abuse trauma: Theory and treatment of the lasting effects.* Newbury Park, CA: Sage.

Briere, J. (1992b). Methodological issues in the study of sexual abuse effects. *Journal of Consulting and Clinical Psychology, 60,* 196–203.

Briere, J. (1992c). Medical symptoms, health risk, and history of childhood sexual abuse [Editorial]. *Mayo Clinic Proceedings, 67,* 603–604.

Briere, J. (1995a). Science versus politics in the delayed memory debate: A commentary. *The Counseling Psychologist, 23,* 290–293.

Briere, J. (1995b). *Trauma Symptom Inventory professional manual.* Odessa, FL: Psychological Assessment Resources.

Briere, J. (1996). A self-trauma model for treating adult survivors of severe child abuse. In Briere, J., Berliner, L., Bulkley, J., Jenny, C., & Reid, T. (Eds.), *The APSAC handbook on child maltreatment.* Newbury Park, CA: Sage.

Briere, J. (in press, a). *Psychological assessment of adult posttraumatic states.* Washington, DC: American Psychological Association.

Briere, J. (in press, b). Psychological assessment of child abuse effects in adults. In J. P. Wilson & T. M. Keane (Eds.), *Assessing psychological trauma and PTSD: A handbook for practitioners.* New York: Guilford.

Briere, J., & Conte, J. (1989, October). *Variables associated with the victim-to-perpetrator transformation.* Paper presented at the Eighth National Conference on Child Abuse and Neglect, Salt Lake City, UT.

Briere, J., & Conte, J. (1993). Self-reported amnesia for abuse in adults molested as children. *Journal of Traumatic Stress, 6,* 21–31.

Briere, J., Elliott, D. M., Harris, K., & Cotman (1995). Trauma Symptom Inventory: Psychometrics and association with childhood and adult trauma in clinical samples. *Journal of Interpersonal Violence, 10,* 387–401.

Briere, J., Evans, D., Runtz, M., & Wall, T. (1988). Symptomatology in men who were molested as children: A comparison study. *American Journal of Orthopsychiatry, 58,* 457–461.

Briere, J., Henschel, D., Smiljanich, K., & Morlan-Magallanes, M. (1990, April). *Self-injurious behavior and child abuse history in adult men and women*. Paper presented at the National Symposium on Child Victimization, Atlanta, Georgia.

Briere, J., & P. A. R. (Psychological Assessment Resources) staff (1995). *Trauma Symptom Inventory scoring program*. Odessa, FL: Psychological Assessment Resources.

Briere, J., & Runtz, M. (1986). Suicidal thoughts and behaviors in former sexual abuse victims. *Canadian Journal of Behavioural Sciences, 18,* 413–423.

Briere, J., & Runtz, M. (1987). Post sexual abuse trauma: Data and implications for clinical practice. *Journal of Interpersonal Violence 2,* 367–379.

Briere, J., & Runtz, M. (1988a). Symptomatology associated with childhood sexual victimization in a non-clinical adult sample. *Child Abuse & Neglect, 12,* 51–59.

Briere, J., & Runtz, M. (1988b). Multivariate correlates of childhood psychological and physical maltreatment among university women. *Child Abuse & Neglect, 12,* 331–341.

Briere, J., & Runtz, M. (1988c). Post sexual abuse trauma. In G. E. Wyatt & G. Powell (Eds.), *The lasting effects of child sexual abuse*. Newbury Park, CA: Sage.

Briere, J., & Runtz, M. (1989a). University males' sexual interest in children: Predicting potential indices of "pedophilia" in a non-forensic sample. *Child Abuse & Neglect, 13,* 65–75.

Briere, J., & Runtz, M. (1989b). The Trauma Symptom Checklist (TSC-33): Early data on a new scale. *Journal of Interpersonal Violence, 4,* 151–163.

Briere, J., & Runtz, M. (1990a). Augmenting Hopkins SCL scales to measure dissociative symptoms: Data from two non-clinical samples. *Journal of Personality Assessment, 55,* 376–379.

Briere, J., & Runtz, M. (1990b). Differential adult symptomatology associated with three types of child abuse histories. *Child Abuse & Neglect: The International Journal, 14,* 357–364.

Briere, J., & Runtz, M. (1993). Child sexual abuse: Long-term sequelae and implications for assessment. *Journal of Interpersonal Violence, 8,* 312–330.

Briere, J., & Smiljanich, K. (1993, August). *Child sexual abuse and subsequent sexual aggression against adult women*. Paper presented at the annual meeting of the American Psychological Association, Toronto, Canada.

Briere, J., Smiljanich, K., & Henschel, D. (1994). Sexual fantasies, gender, and molestation history. *Child Abuse & Neglect, 18,* 131–137.

Briere, J., Ward, R., & Hartsough, W. R. (1983). Sex typing and cross-sex typing in "androgynous" subjects. *Journal of Personality Assessment, 47,* 300–302.

Briere, J., & Zaidi, L. Y. (1989). Sexual abuse histories and sequelae in female psychiatric emergency room patients. *American Journal of Psychiatry, 146,* 1602–1606.

Browne, A., & Finkelhor, D. (1986a). Impact of child sexual abuse: A review of the research. *Psychological Bulletin, 99,* 66–77.

Browne, A., & Finkelhor, D. (1986b). Initial and long-term effects: A review of the research. In D. Finkelhor, (Ed.) *A sourcebook on child sexual abuse.* Beverly Hills, CA: Sage.

Brownmiller, S. (1975). *Against our will: Men, women, and rape.* New York: Simon & Schuster.

Burgess, A. W., & Grant, C. A. (1988). *Children traumatized in sex rings.* Washington, DC: National Center for Missing and Exploited Children.

Burgess, A. W., & Holmstrom, L. L. (1974). Rape trauma syndrome. *American Journal of Psychiatry, 131,* 981–986.

Burt, M. R. (1980). Cultural myths and supports for rape. *Journal of Personality and Social Psychology, 38,* 217–230.

Butcher, J. N., Dahlstrom, W. G., Graham, J. R., Tellegen, A., & Kaemmer, B. (1989). *Minnesota Multiphasic Personality Inventory (MMPI-2): Manual for administration and scoring.* Minneapolis: University of Minnesota Press.

Butler, S. (1978). *Conspiracy of silence: The trauma of incest.* San Francisco: Volcano Press.

Byrne, D. (1961). The repression-sensitization scale: Rationale, reliability, and validity. *Journal of Personality, 29,* 334–339.

Campbell, R. J. (1989). *Psychiatric dictionary* (6th ed.) New York: Oxford University Press.

Caplan, P. J., & Hall-McCorquodale, I. (1985). Mother-blaming in major clinical journals. *American Journal of Orthopsychiatry, 55,* 345–353.

Chu, J. A., & Dill, D. L. (1990). Dissociative symptoms in relation to childhood physical and sexual abuse. *American Journal of Psychiatry, 147,* 887–892.

Classen, C. (Ed.) (1995). *Treating women molested in childhood.* San Francisco: Jossey Bass.

Coates, D., & Winston, T. (1983). Counteracting the deviance of depression: Peer support groups for victims. *Journal of Social Issues, 39,* 169–194.

Cole, C. L. (1985). A group design for adult female survivors of childhood incest. *Women and Therapy, 4,* 71–82.

Cole, C. H., & Barney, E. E. (1987). Safeguards and the therapeutic window: A group treatment strategy for adult incest survivors. *American Journal of Orthopsychiatry, 57,* 601–609.

Cole, P. M., & Putnam, F. W. (1992). Effect of incest on self and social functioning: A developmental psychopathology perspective. *Journal of Consulting and Clinical Psychology, 60,* 174–184.

Conte, J., & Schuerman, J. R. (1987). The effects of sexual abuse on children: A multidimensional view. *Journal of Interpersonal Violence, 2,* 380–390.

Coons, P. M., & Milstein, V. (1986). Psychosexual disturbances in multiple personality: Characteristics, etiology, and treatment. *Journal of Clinical Psychiatry, 47,* 106–110.

Corne, S., Briere, J., & Esses, L. (1992). Women's attitudes and fantasies about rape as a function of early exposure to pornography. *Journal of Interpersonal Violence, 4,* 454–461.

Cornell, W. F., & Olio, K. A. (1991). Integrating affect in treatment with adult survivors of physical and sexual abuse. *American Journal of Orthopsychiatry, 61,* 59–69.

Courtois, C. A. (1979a). *Characteristics of a volunteer sample of adult women who experienced incest in childhood or adolescence.* Unpublished doctoral dissertation, University of Maryland.

Courtois, C. A. (1979b). The incest experience and its aftermath. *Victimology: An International Journal, 4,* 337–347.

Courtois, C. A. (1988). *Healing the incest wound: adult survivors in therapy.* New York: W.W. Norton.

Courtois, C. A. (1991). Theory, sequencing, and strategy in treating adult survivors. In J. Briere (Ed.), *Treating victims of child sexual abuse* (pp. 47–60). San Francisco: Jossey-Bass.

Courtois, C. (1995). Walking a fine line: Issues in the assessment and diagnosis of women molested in childhood. In C. Classen (Ed.), *Treating women molested in childhood.* San Francisco: Jossey-Bass.

Courtois, C. A., & Leehan, J. (1982, May). Group treatment for grown-up abused children. *The Personnel and Guidance Journal,* 564–567.

Davidson, H. A., & Loken, G. A. (1987). *Child pornography and prostitution: Background and legal analysis.* Washington, DC: National Center for Missing and Exploited Children.

DeFrancis, V. (1969). *Protecting the child victim of sex crimes committed by adults.* Denver: American Humane Association.

Demaré, D., & Briere, J. (1994, August). *Childhood maltreatment and current symptomatology in 1,179 university students.* Paper presented at the annual meeting of the American Psychological Association, Los Angeles, CA.

Demaré, D., Briere, J., & Lips, H. M. (1988). Violent pornography and self-reported likelihood of sexual aggression. *Journal of Research in Personality, 22,* 140–153.

Dembo, R., Williams, L., LaVoie, L., Barry, E., Getreu, A., Wish, E., Schmeider, J., & Washburn, M. (1989). Physical abuse, sexual victimization, and illicit drug use: Replication of a structural analysis among a new sample of high-risk youths. *Violence and Victims, 4,* 121–138.

DeYoung, M. (1981). Case reports: The sexual exploitation of incest victims by health professionals. *Victimology, 6,* 92–101.

Donaldson, M. A., & Gardner, R. (1985). Diagnosis and treatment of traumatic stress among women after childhood incest. In C. Figley (Ed.), *Trauma and its wake.* New York: Brunner/Mazel.

Drauker, C. D. (1992). *Counseling survivors of childhood sexual abuse.* Newbury Park: Sage.

Drossman, D. A., Lesserman, J., Nachman, G., Li, Z., Gluck, H., Toomey, T. C., Mitchell, C. M. (1990). Sexual and physical abuse in women with functional or organic gastrointestinal disorders. *Annuals of Internal Medicine, 113,* 828–833.

Elliott, D. M. (1994a). Impaired object relations in professional women molested as children. *Psychotherapy, 31,* 79–86.

Elliott, D. M. (1994b). Assessing adult victims of interpersonal violence. In J. Briere (Ed.), *Assessing and treating victims of violence.* San Francisco: Jossey-Bass.

Elliott, D. M., & Briere, J. (1992). Sexual abuse trauma among professional women: Validating the Trauma Symptom Checklist–40 (TSC-40). *Child Abuse & Neglect, 16,* 391–398.

Elliott, D. M., & Briere, J. (1994). Forensic sexual abuse evaluations of older children: Disclosures and symptomatology. *Behavioral Sciences and the Law, 12,* 261–277.

Elliott, D. M., & Briere, J. (1995). Transference and countertransference. In C. Clausen (Ed.), *Treating women molested in childhood.* San Fransisco: Jossey Bass.

Elliott, D. M., & Briere, J. (1995). Posttraumatic stress associated with delayed recall of sexual abuse: A general population study. *Journal of Traumatic Stress, 8,* 629–647.

Elliott, D. M., & Guy, J. D. (1993). Mental health professionals versus non-mental-health professionals: Childhood trauma and adult functioning. *Professional Psychology: Research and Practice, 24,* 83–90.

Elliott, D. M., & Mok, D. (1995, April). *Adult sexual assault: Prevalence, symptomatology, and sex differences.* Paper presented at the annual meeting of the Western Psychological Association, San Francisco, CA.

Enns, C. Z., McNeilly, C. L., Corkery, J. M., & Gilbert, M. S. (1995). The debate about delayed memories of child sexual abuse: A feminist perspective. *The Counseling Psychologist, 23,* 181–279.

Feldman-Summers, S., & Pope, K. S. (1994). The experience of "forgetting" childhood abuse: A national survey of psychologists. *Journal of Consulting and Clinical Psychology, 62,* 636–639.

Finkelhor, D. (1979a). *Sexually victimized children.* New York: Free Press.

Finkelhor, D. (1979b). What's wrong with sex between adults and children. *American Journal of Orthopsychiatry, 49,* 692–697.

Finkelhor, D. (1980). Risk factors in the sexual victimization of children. Child Abuse & Neglect, 4, 265–273.

Finkelhor, D. (1984). *Child sexual abuse: New theory and research.* New York: Free Press.

Finkelhor, D. (1987). The trauma of child sexual abuse: Two models. *Journal of Interpersonal Violence, 2,* 348–366.

Finkelhor, D. (1990). Early and long-term effects of child sexual abuse: An update. *Professional Psychology: Research and Practice, 21,* 325–330.

Finkelhor, D., Araji, S., Baron, L., Browne, A., Peters, S. D., & Wyatt, G. E. (1986). *A sourcebook on child sexual abuse.* Newbury Park, CA: Sage.

Finkelhor, D., & Browne, A. (1985). The traumatic impact of child sexual abuse: A conceptualization. *American Journal of Orthopsychiatry, 55,* 530–541.

Finkelhor, D., Hotaling, G., Lewis, I. A., & Smith, C. (1989). Sexual abuse and its relationship to later sexual satisfaction, marital status, religion, and attitudes. *Journal of Interpersonal Violence, 4,* 279–399.

Fisher, P. M. (1991). *Women survivors of childhood sexual abuse: Clinical sequelae and treatment.* Unpublished doctoral dissertation, Simon Fraser University, Burnaby, British Columbia.

Foa, E. B., Riggs, D. S., Dancu, C. V., Rothbaum, B. O. (1993). Reliability and validity of a brief instrument assessing post-traumatic stress disorder. *Journal of Traumatic Stress, 6,* 459–474.

Foa, E. B., Rothbaum, B. O., Riggs, D. S., & Murdock, T. B. (1991). Treatment of posttraumatic disorder in rape victims: A comparison between cognitive-behavioral procedures and counseling. *Journal of Consulting and Clinical Psychology, 59,* 715–723.

Follette, V. M. (1991). Marital therapy for sexual abuse survivors. In J. Briere (Ed.), *Treating victims of child sexual abuse.* San Francisco: Jossey-Bass.

Follette, V. M., & Pistorello, J. (1995). Couples therapy. In C. Classen (Ed.), *Treating women molested in childhood.* San Francisco: Jossey-Bass.

Foy, D. W., Sipprelle, R. C., Rueger, D. B., & Carroll, E. M. (1984). Etiology of posttraumatic stress syndrome in Vietnam veterans: Analysis of premilitary, military, and combat exposure influences. *Journal of Consulting and Clinical Psychology, 52,* 79–87.

Frank, E., & Stewart, B. D. (1983). Depressive symptoms in rape victims: A revisit. *Journal of Affective Disorders, 7,* 77–85.

Freud, S. (1958/1900). The interpretation of dreams. In J. Strachey (Ed. and Trans.), *The complete psychological works of Sigmund Freud* (stand. ed.). London: Hogarth.

Friedrich, W. N. (1994). Assessing children for the effects of sexual victimization. In J. Briere (Ed.), *Assessing and treating victims of violence* (New Directions for Mental Health Services Series [MHS No. 64]). San Francisco: Jossey-Bass.

Friedrich, W. N. (1995). *Treatment of sexually abused boys.* Newbury Park, CA: Sage.

Friedrich, W. N. (1996). An integrated model of therapy for abused children. In J. Briere, L. Berliner, J. Bulkley, C. Jenny, & T. Reid (Eds.), *The APSAC handbook on child maltreatment.* Newbury Park, CA: Sage.

Friedrich, W. N., Beilke, R. L., & Urquiza, A. J. (1987). Children from sexually abusive families: A behavioral comparison. *Journal of Interpersonal Violence, 2,* 391–402.

Fromuth, M. E. (1985). The relationship of child sexual abuse with later psychological and sexual adjustment in a sample of college women. *Child Abuse & Neglect, 10,* 5–15.

Gardner, R. (1992). *True and false accusations of child sexual abuse.* Cresskill, NJ: Creative Therapeutics.

Gebhard, P., Gagnon, J., Pomeroy, W., & Christenson, C. (1965). *Sex offenders: An analysis of types.* New York: Harper & Row.

Gelinas, D. J. (1981). Identification and treatment of incest victims. In E. Howell and M. Bayes (Eds.), *Women and mental health.* New York: Basic Books.

Gelinas, D. J. (1983). The persisting negative effects of incest. *Psychiatry, 46,* 312–333.

Gil, E. (1988). *Treatment of adult survivors of childhood abuse.* Rockville, MD: Launch Press.

Gil, E., & Briere, G. (1995, August). *Self-mutilation: Incidence, correlates, and self-reported effects.* Paper presented at the annual meeting of the American Psychological Association, New York, NY.

Gold, E. R. (1986). Long-term effects of sexual victimization in childhood: An attributional approach. *Journal of Consulting and Clinical Psychology, 54,* 471–475.

Gold, S. R., Milan, L. D., Mayall, A., & Johnson, A. E. (1994). A cross-validation study of the Trauma Symptom Checklist: The role of mediating variables. *Journal of interpersonal Violence, 9,* 12–26.

Goodman, B., & Nowak-Scibelli, D. (1985). Group treatment for women incestuously abused as children. *International Journal of Group Psychotherapy, 54,* 531–544.

Goodwin, J. (1984). Incest victims exhibit Post Traumatic Stress Disorder. *Clinical Psychiatry News, 12,* 13.

Goodwin, J., Simms, M., & Bergman, R. (1979). Hysterical seizures: A sequel to incest. *American Journal of Orthopsychiatry, 49,* 698–703.

Gordy, P. L. (1983, May). Group work that supports adult victims of childhood incest. *Social Casework,* 300–307.

Greenwald, E., & Leitenberg, H. (1990). Post-traumatic stress disorder in a nonclinical and nonstudent sample of adult women sexually abused as children. *Journal of Interpersonal Violence, 5,* 217–228.

Gross, M. (1979). Incestuous rape: A cause for hysterical seizures in four adolescent girls. *American Journal of Orthopsychiatry, 49,* 704–708.

Gross, R. J., Doerr, H., Caldirola, D., Guzinski, G. M., & Ripley, H. S. (1980–81). Borderline syndrome and incest in chronic pain patients. *International Journal of Psychiatry in Medicine, 10,* 79–98.

Groves, J. E. (1975). Management of the borderline patient on a medical or surgical ward: The psychiatric consultant's role. *International Journal of Psychiatry in Medicine, 6,* 337–348.

Gunderson, J. G., & Singer, M. T. (1975). Defining borderline patients: An overview. *American Journal of Psychiatry, 132,* 1–10.

Haber, J., & Roos, C. (1985). Effects of spouse abuse and/or sexual abuse in the development and maintenance of chronic pain in women. In H. L. Fields et al. (Eds.), *Advances in pain research and therapy* (Vol. 9). New York: Raven.

Hart, S. N., & Brassard, M. R. (1987). A major threat to children's mental health: Psychological maltreatment. *American Psychologist, 42,* 160–165.

Harter, S., Alexander, P., & Neimeyer, R. (1988). Long-term effects of incestuous child abuse in college women: Social adjustment, social cognition, and family characteristics. *Journal of Consulting and Clinical Psychology, 54,* 466–470.

Hartmann, E. (1984). *The nightmare: The psychology and biology of terrifying dreams.* New York: Basic Books.

Henderson J. (1975). Incest. In A. M. Freedman, H. L. Kaplan, & B. S. Sadock (Eds.), *Comprehensive textbook of psychiatry.* Baltimore: Williams & Wilkins.

Henderson, J. (1983). Is incest harmful? *Canadian Journal of Psychiatry, 28,* 34–39.

Herman, J. L. (1981). *Father-daughter incest.* Cambridge: Harvard University Press.

Herman, J. L. (1986). Histories of violence in an outpatient population. *American Journal of Psychiatry, 56,* 137–141.

Herman, J. L. (1992). *Trauma and recovery: The aftermath of violence—from domestic abuse to political terror.* New York: Basic Books.

Herman, J. L., Perry, C., & van der Kolk, B. A. (1989). Childhood trauma in borderline personality disorder. *American Journal of Psychiatry, 146,* 490–494.

Herman, J. L., Russell, D. E. H., & Trocki, K. (1986). Long-term effects of incestuous abuse in childhood. *American Journal of Psychiatry, 143,* 1293–1296.

Herman, J. L., & Schatzow, E. (1984). Time-limited group therapy for women with a history of incest. *International Journal of Group Psychotherapy, 34,* 605–616.

Herman, J. L., & Schatzow, E. (1987). Recovery and verification of memories of childhood sexual trauma. *Psychoanalytic Psychology, 4,* 1–4.

Herman, J. L., & van der Kolk, B. A. (1987). Traumatic antecedents of borderline personality disorder. In B. A. van der Kolk (Ed.), *Psychological trauma.* Washington, DC: American Psychiatric Press.

Holroyd, J. C., & Brodsky, A. M. (1977). Psychologists' attitudes and practices regarding erotic and nonerotic physical contact with patients. *American Psychologist, 32,* 843–849.

Horowitz, M. D., Wilner, N., & Alvarez, W. (1979). Impacts of Event Scale: A measure of subjective stress. *Psychosomatic Medicine, 41,* 209–218.

Horowitz, M. J. (1976). *Stress response syndromes.* New York: Jason Aronson.

Horowitz, M. J. (1986). Stress-response syndromes: A review of posttraumatic and adjustment disorders. *Hospital and Community Psychiatry, 37,* 241–249.

Hunter, J. A. (1991). A comparison of the psychosocial maladjustment of adult males and females sexually molested as children. *Journal of Interpersonal Violence, 6,* 205–217.

James, J., & Meyerding, J. (1977). Early sexual experience and prostitution. *American Journal of Psychiatry, 134,* 1381–1385.

Janoff-Bulman, B. (1992). *Shattered assumptions: Towards a new psychology of trauma.* New York: Free Press.

Janoff-Bulman, R., & Frieze, I. H. (1983). A theoretical perspective for understanding reactions to victimization. *Journal of Social Issues, 39,* 1–17.

Jehu, D. (1989). *Beyond sexual abuse: Therapy with women who were childhood victims.* New York: Wiley.

Jehu, D., & Gazan, M. (1983). Psychosocial adjustment of women who were sexually victimized in childhood or adolescence. *Canadian Journal of Community Mental Health, 2,* 71–82.

Jehu, D., Gazan, M., & Klassen, C. (1984–85). Common therapeutic targets among women who were sexually abused in childhood. *Journal of Social Work and Human Sexuality, 3,* 25–45.

Jehu, D., Klassen, C., & Gazan, M. (1985–86). Cognitive restructuring of distorted beliefs associated with childhood sexual abuse. *Journal of Social Work and Human Sexuality, 4,* 1–35.

Johanek, M. F. (1988). Treatment of male victims of child sexual abuse in military service. In S. M. Sgroi, *Vulnerable populations* (Vol. 1). Lexington, MA: Lexington Books.

Johnson, R. L., & Shrier, D. (1987) Past sexual victimization by females of male patients in an adolescent medicine clinic population. *American Journal of Psychiatry, 244,* 650–652.

Keane, T. M., Fairbank, J. A., Caddell, J. M., Zimering, R. T., Taylor, K. L., & Mora, C. A. (1989). Clinical evaluation of a measure to assess combat exposure. *Psychological Assessment, 1,* 53–55.

Kelly, S. J. (1996). Ritualistic abuse of children. In J. Briere, L. Berliner, J. Bulkley, C. Jenny, & T. Reid (Eds.). *APSAC Handbook on Child Maltreatment.* Newbury Park, CA: Sage.

Kelly, R. J., MacDonald, V. M., & Waterman, J. M. (1987, January). *Psychological symptomatology in adult male victims of child sexual abuse: A preliminary report.* Paper presented at the joint conference of the American Psychological Association, Division 12, and the Hawaii Psychological Association, Honolulu, Hawaii.

Kernberg, O. F. (1975). *Borderline conditions and pathological narcissism.* New York: Jason Aronson.

Kluft, R. P. (1990). Incest and subsequent revictimization: The case of therapist-patient sexual exploitation, with a description of the Sitting Duck Syndrome. In R. P. Kluft (Ed.), *Incest-related syndromes of adult psychopathology.* Washington, DC: American Psychiatric Press.

Koss, M. P., & Harvey, M. R. (1991). *The rape victim.* Newbury Park: Sage.

Kroll, J. (1993). *PTSD/borderlines in therapy: Finding the balance.* New York: Norton.

Krystal, H. (1978). Trauma and affects. *Psychoanalytic Study of the Child, 33,* 81–116.

Lamb, F. (1986). Treating sexually abused children: Issues of blame and responsibility. *American Journal of Orthopsychiatry, 56,* 303–307.

Langevin, R., Handy, L., Hook, H., Day, D., & Russon, A. (1985). Are incestuous fathers pedophilic and aggressive? In R. Langevin (Ed.), *Erotic preference, gender identity, and aggression.* New York: Erlbaum.

Lanktree, C. B. (1994). Treating child victims of sexual abuse. In J. Briere (Ed.), *Assessing and treating victims of violence* (New Directions for Mental Health Services Series [MHS No. 64]). San Francisco: Jossey-Bass.

Lanktree, C. B., Briere, J., & Zaidi, L. Y. (1991). Incidence and impacts of sexual abuse in a child outpatient sample: The role of direct inquiry. *Child Abuse & Neglect, 15*, 447–453.

Lerman, H. (1986). *A mote in Freud's eye: From psychoanalysis to the psychology of women.* New York: Springer.

Lerner, M. J. (1980). *The belief in a just world: A fundamental delusion.* New York: Plenum Press.

Lindberg, F. H., & Distad, L. J. (1985a). Post-traumatic stress disorders in women who experienced childhood incest. *Child Abuse & Neglect, 9,* 329–334.

Lindberg, F. H., & Distad, L. J. (1985b) Survival responses to incest: Adolescents in crisis. *Child Abuse & Neglect, 9,* 521–526.

Lindsay, D. S. (1995). Beyond backlash: Comments on Enns, McNeilly, Corkery, and Gilbert. *The Counseling Psychologist, 23,* 280–289.

Linehan, M. M. (1993). *Cognitive-behavioral treatment of borderline personality disorder.* New York: Guilford.

Lobel, C. M. (1990). *Relationship between childhood sexual abuse and borderline personality disorder in women psychiatric inpatients.* Unpublished doctoral dissertation, California Graduate Institute, Los Angeles, CA.

Lipovsky, J. A., Saunders, B. E., & Murphy, S. M. (1989). Depression, anxiety, and behavior problems among victims of father-child sexual assault and nonabused siblings. *Journal of Interpersonal Violence, 4,* 452–468.

Loftus, E. F. (1993). The reality of repressed memories. *American Psychologist, 48,* 518–537.

Loftus, E. F. & Ketcham, K. (1994). *The myth of repressed memory: False memories and allegations of sexual abuse.* New York: St. Martin's Press.

Loftus, E. F., Polonsky, S., & Fullilove, M. T. (1994). Memories of childhood sexual abuse: Remembering and repressing. *Psychology of Women Quarterly, 18,* 67–84.

Lubell, D., & Soong, W. (1982). Group therapy with sexually abused adolescents. *Canadian Journal of Psychiatry, 27,* 311–315.

Lynn, S. J., & Rhue, J. W. (1988). Fantasy proneness: Hypnosis, developmental antecedents, and psychopathology. *American Psychologist, 43,* 35–44.

Magana, D. (1990). *The impact of client-therapist sexual intimacy and child sexual abuse on psychosexual and psychological functioning.* Unpublished doctoral dissertation, University of California at Los Angeles, Los Angeles, California.

Malamuth, N. M. (1981). Rape proclivity among males. *Journal of Social Issues, 37,* 138–157.

Malamuth, N. M., & Briere, J. (1986). Sexual violence in the media: Indirect effects on aggression against women. *Journal of Social Issues, 42,* 75–92.

Maltz, W. (1988). Identifying and treating the sexual repercussions of incest: A couples therapy approach. *Journal of Sex and Marital Therapy, 14,* 145–163.

Maltz, W., & Holman, B. (1987) *Incest and sexuality: A guide to understanding and healing.* Lexington, MA: Lexington Books.

Masson, J. M. (1984). *The assault on truth: Freud's suppression of the seduction theory.* New York: Farrar, Straus & Giroux.

Masterson, J. F. (1976). *Psychotherapy with the borderline adult.* New York: Brunner/Mazel.

McAnarney, E. (1975). The older abused child. *Pediatrics, 55,* 298–299

McCann, I. L., & Pearlman, L. A. (1990). *Psychological trauma and the adult survivor: Theory, therapy, and transformation.* New York: Brunner/Mazel.

McCann, L., Pearlman, L. A., Sackheim, D. K., & Abramson, D. J. (1985). Assessment and treatment of the adult survivor of childhood sexual abuse within a schema framework. In S. M. Sgroi (Ed.), *Vulnerable populations* (Vol. 1). Lexington, MA: Lexington Books.

McCord, J. (1985). Long-term adjustment in female survivors of incest: An exploratory study. *Dissertation Abstracts International, 46,* 650B.

McCormack, A., Janus, M. D., & Burgess, A. W. (1986). Runaway youths and sexual victimization: Gender differences in an adolescent runaway population. *Child Abuse & Neglect, 10,* 387–395.

McLeer, S. V., Deblinger, E., Atkins, M. S., Foa, E. B., & Ralphe, D. L. (1988). Posttraumatic stress disorder in sexually abused children. *Journal of the American Academy of Child and Adolescent Psychiatry, 27,* 650–654.

Meiselman, K. C. (1978). *Incest: A psychological study of causes and effects with treatment recommendations.* San Francisco: Jossey Bass.

Meiselman, K. C. (1990). *Resolving the trauma of incest: Reintegration therapy with survivors.* San Francisco: Jossey-Bass.

Meiselman, K. C. (1994). Treating survivors of child sexual abuse: A strategy for reintegration. In J. Briere (Ed.), *Assessing and treating victims of violence* (New Directions for Mental Health Services series [MHS No. 64]). San Francisco: Jossey-Bass.

Mendel, M. P. (1995). *The male survivor: The impact of sexual abuse.* Thousand Oaks, CA: Sage.

Miller, A. (1984). *Thou shalt not be aware: Society's betrayal of the child.* New York: Meridian.

Miller, B. A., Downs, W. R., Gondoli, D. M., & Keil, A. (1987). The role of childhood sexual abuse in the development of alcoholism in women. *Violence and Victims, 2,* 157–172.

Miller, D. T., & Porter, C. A. (1983). Self-blame in victims of violence. *Journal of Social Issues, 39,* 139–152.

Millon, T. (1994). *Manual for the MCMI-III.* Minneapolis: National Computer Systems.

Morey, L. C. (1991). Personality Assessment Inventory: Professional manual. Odessa, FL: Psychological Assessment Resources.

Morrison, J. (1989). Childhood sexual histories of women with somatization disorder. *American Journal of Psychiatry, 146,* 239–241.

Murphy, S. M., Kilpatrick, D. G., Amick-McMullan, A., Veronen, L. J., Paduhovich, J., Best, C. L., Villeponteaux, L. A., &. Saunders, B. E. (1988). Current psychological functioning of child sexual assault survivors: A community study. *Journal of Interpersonal Violence, 3,* 55–79.

Neumann, D. A., Houskamp, B. M., Pollock, V. E., & Briere, J. (1996). The long-term sequelae of childhood sexual abuse in women: A meta-analytic review. *Child Maltreatment, 1,* 6–16.

NiCarthy, G., Merriam, K., & Coffman, S. (1984). *Talking it out: A guide to groups for abused women.* Seattle: Seal Press.

Ofshe, R., & Watters, E. (1994). *Making monsters: False memories, psychotherapy, and sexual hysteria.* New York: Scribners.

Ogata, S. N., Silk, K. R., Goodrich, S., Lohr, N. E., Westen, D., & Hill, E. M. (1990). Childhood sexual and physical abuse in adult patients with borderline personality disorder. *American Journal of Psychiatry, 147,* 1008–1013.

Olio, K. A., & Cornell, W. F. (1993). The therapeutic relationship as the foundation for treatment with adult survivors of sexual abuse. *Psychotherapy, 30,* 512–523.

Owens, T. H. (1984). Personality traits of female psychotherapy patients with a history of incest: A research note. *Journal of Personality Assessment, 48,* 606–608.

Ounce of Prevention Fund. (1987). *Child sexual abuse: A hidden factor in adolescent sexual behavior.* Chicago, Author.

Paddison, P. L., Einbender, R. G., Maker, E., & Strain, J. J. (1993). Group treatment with incest survivors. In P. L. Paddison (Ed.), *Treatment of adult survivors of incest.* Washington, D.C.: American Psychiatric press.

Paidika. (1993). Interview: Holida Underwager and Ralph Underwager. Paidika: *The Journal of Pedophilia, 3,* 2–12.

Pearlman, L. A., & Saakvitne, K. W. (1995). *Trauma and the therapist: Coun-*

tertransference and vicarious traumatization in psychotherapy with incest survivors. New York: W. W. Norton.

Perloff, L. S. (1983). Perceptions of vulnerability to victimization. *Journal of Social Issues, 39,* 41–61.

Perry, C. J., & Klerman, C. L. (1978). The borderline patient. *Archives of General Psychiatry, 35,* 141–150.

Peters, J. J (1976). Children who are victims of sexual assault and the psychology of offenders. *American Journal of Psychotherapy, 30,* 398–421.

Peters, S. D. (1984). *The relationship between childhood sexual victimization and adult depression among Afro-American and white women.* Unpublished doctoral dissertation, University of California at Los Angeles.

Peters, S. D., Wyatt, G. E., & Finkelhor, D. (1986). Prevalence. In D. Finkelhor, S. Araji, L. Baron, A. Browne, S. D. Peters, & G. E. Wyatt (Eds.), *A sourcebook on child sexual abuse.* Beverly Hills: Sage.

Peterson, C., & Seligman, M. E. P. (1983). Learned helplessness and victimization. *Journal of Social Issues, 39,* 103–116.

Pollock, V. E., Briere, J., Schneider, L., Knop, J., Mednick, S. A., & Goodwin, D. W. (1990). Childhood antecedents of antisocial behavior: Parental alcoholism and physical abusiveness. *American Journal of Psychiatry, 147,* 1290–1293.

Pope, K. S. (1994). *Sexual involvement with therapists: Patient assessment, subsequent therapy, forensics.* Washington, DC: American Psychological Association.

Pope, K. S., & Bouhoutsos, J. C. (1986). *Sexual intimacies between therapists and patients.* New York: Praeger/Greenwood.

Pope, K. S., & Feldman-Summers, S. (1992). National survey of psychologists' sexual and physical abuse history and their evaluation of training and competence in these areas. *Professional Psychology: Research and Practice, 23,* 353–361.

Putnam, F. W. (1989). *Diagnosis and treatment of multiple personality disorder.* New York: Guilford Press.

Rachman, S. (1980). Emotional processing. *Behavior, Research, and Therapy, 18,* 51–60.

Reich, J. W., & Gutierres, S. E. (1979). Escape/aggression incidence in sexually abused juvenile delinquents. *Criminal Justice and Behavior, 6,* 239–243.

Reiker, P. P., & Carmen, E. (1986). The victim-to-patient process: The disconfirmation and transformation of abuse. *American Journal of Orthopsychiatry, 56,* 360–370.

Resick, P. A., & Schnicke, M. K. (1993). *Cognitive processing therapy for rape victims: A treatment manual.* Newbury Park: Sage.

Rinsley, D. B. (1980). *Treatment of the severely disturbed adolescent.* New York: Jason Aronson.

Rogers, M. L. (1992). Evaluating adult litigants who allege injuries from sexual abuse: Clinical assessment methods for traumatic memories. *Issues in Child Abuse Accusations, 4,* 221–238.

Rokous, F., Carter, D., & Prentky, R. (1988, April). *Sexual and physical abuse in the developmental histories of child molesters.* Paper presented at the National Symposium on Child Abuse, Anaheim, CA.

Rosenfeld, A. (1979). Incidence of a history of incest in 18 female psychiatric patients. *American Journal of Psychiatry, 136,* 791–795.

Ross, C. A. (1989). *Multiple personality disorder: Diagnosis, clinical features, and treatment.* New York: Wiley.

Ross, R. R. (1980). Violence in, violence out. Child abuse and self-mutilation in adolescent offenders. *Canadian Journal of Criminology, 22,* 273–287.

Rowan, A. B., Foy, D. W., Rodriguez, N., & Ryan, S. (1994). Posttraumatic stress disorder in a clinical sample of adults sexually abused as children. *Child Abuse & Neglect, 18,* 51–61.

Runtz, M. (1987). *The psychosocial adjustment of women who were sexually and physically abused during childhood and early adulthood: A focus on revictimization.* Unpublished master's thesis, University of Manitoba.

Runtz, M., & Briere, J. (1986). Adolescent "acting out" and childhood history of sexual abuse. *Journal of Interpersonal Violence, 1,* 326–334.

Rush, P. (1980). *The best kept secret: Sexual abuse of children.* Englewood Cliffs, NJ: Prentice Hall.

Russell, D. E. H. (1983a). The prevalence and incidence of forcible rape and attempted rape of females. *Victimology: An International Journal, 7,* 1–4.

Russell, D. E. H. (1983b). The incidence and prevalence of intrafamilial and extrafamilial sexual abuse of female children. *Child Abuse & Neglect, 7,* 133–146.

Russell, D. E. H. (1986). *The secret trauma: Incest in the lives of girls and women.* New York: Basic Books.

Saigh, P. A. (Ed.) (1992). *Posttraumatic stress disorder: A behavioral approach to assessment and treatment.* Needham Heights, MA: Allyn & Bacon.

Salter, (1995). *Transforming trauma: A guide to understanding and treating adult survivors of child sexual abuse.* Newbury Park, CA: Sage.

Saunders, B. E., Villeponteaux, L. A., Lipovsky, J. A., Kilpatrick, D. G., & Veronen, L. J. (1992). Child sexual assault as a risk factor for mental disorders among women: A community survey. *Journal of Interpersonal Violence, 7,* 189–204.

Scott, R. L., & Stone, D. A. (1986). MMPI profile constellations in incest families. *Journal of Consulting and Clinical Psychology, 54,* 364–368.

Sedney, M. A., & Brooks, B. (1984). Factors associated with a history of childhood sexual experiences in a nonclinical female population. *Journal of the American Academy of Child Psychiatry, 23,* 215, 218.

Seligman, M. E. P. (1975). *Helplessness: On depression, development, and death.* San Francisco: W. H. Freeman.

Sgroi, S. M., & Bunk, B. S. (1988). A clinical approach to adult survivors of child sexual abuse. In S. M. Sgroi, *Vulnerable populations* (Vol. 2). Lexington, MA: Lexington Books.

Shay, J. T. (1992). Countertransference in the family therapy of survivors of sexual abuse. *Child Abuse & Neglect, 16,* 585–593.

Silbert, M. H., & Pines, A. M. (1981). Sexual child abuse as an antecedent to prostitution. *Child Abuse & Neglect, 5,* 407–411.

Silver, R. L., Boon, C., & Stones, M. H. (1983). Searching for meaning in misfortune: Making sense of incest. *Journal of Social Issues, 39,* 81–101.

Smiljanich, K., & Briere, J. (1993, August). *Sexual abuse history and trauma symptoms in a university sample.* Paper presented at the annual meeting of the American Psychological Association, Toronto, Canada.

Spence, J. T., & Helmreich, R. (1978). *Psychological dimensions of masculinity and femininity: Their correlates and antecedents.* Austin, TX: University of Texas Press.

Spiegel, H., & Spiegel, D. (1978). *Trance and treatment.* New York: Basic Books.

Springs, F. E., & Friedrich, W. N. (1992). Health risk behaviors and medical sequelae of childhood sexual abuse. *Mayo Clinic Proceedings, 67,* 527–532.

Stein, J. A., Golding, J. M., Siegel, J. M., Burnam, M. A., & Sorenson, S. B. (1988). Long-term psychological sequelae of child sexual abuse: The Los Angeles Epidemiological Catchment Area Study. In G.E. Wyatt, & G. Powell, (Eds.), *The lasting effects of child sexual abuse.* Newbury Park, CA: Sage.

Stukas-Davis, C. (1990). *The influence of childhood sexual abuse and male sex role socialization on adult sexual functioning.* Unpublished doctoral dissertation, California School of Professional Psychology, Los Angeles.

Summit, R. (1983). The child sexual abuse accommodation syndrome. *Child Abuse & Neglect, 7,* 177–193.

Summit, R. (1987, December). *Wingspread briefing paper.* Invited paper presented at the Wingspread Symposium: Child Sexual Abuse—Recommendations for Prevention and Treatment Policy, Racine, WI.

Summit, R. (1988). Hidden victims, hidden pain: Societal avoidance of child sexual abuse. In G. E. Wyatt & G. Powell (Eds.), *The lasting effects of child sexual abuse.* Newbury Park, CA: Sage.

Summit, R., & Kryso, J. (1978) Sexual abuse of children: A clinical spectrum. *American Journal of Orthopsychiatry, 48,* 237–251.

Symonds, M. (1975). Victims of violence: Psychological effects and aftereffects. *The American Journal of Psychoanalysis, 35,* 19–26.

Terr, L. C. (1985). Psychic trauma in children and adolescents. *Psychiatric Clinics of North America, 8,* 815–833.

Tsai, M., Feldman-Summers, S., & Edgar, M. (1979). Childhood molestation: Variables related to differential impacts on psychosexual functioning in adult women. *Journal of Abnormal Psychology, 88,* 407–417.

Tsai, M., & Wagner, N. N. (1978). Therapy groups for women sexually molested as children. *Archives of Sexual Behavior, 7,* 417–427.

Urquiza, A. J., & Crowley, C. (1986, May). *Sex differences in the survivors of childhood sexual abuse.* Paper presented at the Fourth National Conference on the Sexual Victimization of Children, New Orleans, LA.

van der Kolk, B. (1987). The psychological consequences of overwhelming life experience. In B. van der Kolk (Ed.), *Psychological trauma.* Washington, DC: American Psychiatric Press.

van der Kolk, B. A. (1994). The body keeps the score: Memory and the evolving psychobiology of posttraumatic stress. *Harvard Review of Psychiatry, 1,* 253–265.

van der Kolk, B. A., Perry, J. C., & Herman, J. L. (1991). Childhood origins of self-destructive behavior. *American Journal of Psychiatry, 146,* 490–494.

Waldinger, R. J. (1987). Intensive psychodynamic therapy with borderline patients: An overview. *American Journal of Psychiatry, 144,* 267–274.

Walker, E., Katon, W., Harrop-Griffiths, I., Holm, L., Russo, I., & Hickok, L. R. (1988). Relationship of chronic pelvic pain to psychiatric diagnoses and childhood sexual abuse. *American Journal of Psychiatry, 145,* 75–80.

Walker, L. E. (1979). *The battered woman.* New York: Harper & Row.

Walsh, B. W., & Rosen, P. (1988). *Self-mutilation: Theory, research, and treatment.* New York: Guilford Press.

Wheeler, R. J., & Berliner, L. (1988). Treating the effects of sexual abuse on children. In G. E. Wyatt & G. Powell (Eds.), *The lasting effects of child sexual abuse.* Newbury Park, CA: Sage.

Widom, C. S. (1989). The cycle of violence. *Science, 244,* 160–166.

Williams, L. M. (1994). Recall of childhood trauma: A prospective study of women's memories of child sexual abuse. *Journal of Consulting and Clinical Psychology, 62,* 1167–1176.

Wirtz, P., & Harrell, A. (1987). Effects of post-assault exposure to attack-similar stimuli on long-term recovery of victims. *Journal of Consulting and Clinical Psychology, 55,* 10–16.

Wolpe, J. (1958). *Psychotherapy by reciprocal inhibition.* Stanford: Stanford university Press.

Woo, R., & Briere, J. (1992, October). *Victimization history and social-psychological problems in female psychiatric emergency room patients.* International Society for Traumatic Stress Studies, Los Angeles, CA.

Wortman, C. B. (1976). Causal attributions and personal control. In J. Harvey, W. J. Ickes, & R. F. Kidd (Eds.), *New directions in attribution research.* Hillsdale, NJ: Erlbaum.

Wyatt, G. E. (1985). The sexual abuse of Afro-American and white American women in childhood. *Child Abuse & Neglect, 9,* 231–240.

Wyatt, G. E., & Mickey, M. R. (1987). Ameliorating the effects of child sexual abuse: An exploratory study of support by parents and others. *Journal of Interpersonal Violence, 2,* 403–414.

Wyatt, G. E., Newcombe, M. D., & Riederle, M. H. (1993). *Sexual abuse and consensual sex: Women's developmental patterns and outcomes.* Newbury Park, CA: Sage.

Yalom, I. (1975). *Theory and practice of group psychotherapy.* New York: Basic Books.

Yama, M. F., Tovey, S. L., Fogas, B. S. (1993). Childhood family environment and sexual abuse as predictors of anxiety and depression in adult women. *American Journal of Orthopsychiatry, 63,* 136–141.

Index

Abreactive techniques in therapy,
132–133
Abuse dichotomy, 56
Abusers
childhood history of, 22
stigmatization by, 16, 56, 86, 135
Acting in, 23
Acting out, 21, 28–32, 68
in group therapy, 172, 179
by males, 187
in severe abuse, 162
by therapists, 49
in therapy, 80, 82
Adaptive behavior
and interpersonal effects of abuse,
22–32
patterns of perception in, 52–71
Adolescence, prostitution in, 27, 55
Adversariality
in interpersonal relations, 27–28
in therapy, 81
Affect
in borderline personality disorder,
42
dread of, 120
in hysteria, 37

modulation and tolerance of, 66,
125–128
dissociation affecting, 139–140
gender differences in, 186, 187, 190
in posttraumatic stress disorder, 7
Age
of abused children and abusers, 8
at critical trauma, and borderline
behavior, 45
of therapists, 91
Aggressive behavior
by abuse survivors, 22, 29
and male sexuality, 184, 185, 187
Alcohol abuse. *See* Substance abuse
Alienation, 22, 28
Ambivalence
in hysteria, 37
in reactions to abuse, 23–24, 28
in seductive behavior, 98
Amnesia
dissociative, 12, 61–64
in sadistic abuse, 158
postsession, in therapy, 143
Anger, 21–22
in borderline personality disorder,
42

EMPOWERING AND HEALING THE BATTERED WOMAN

A Model for Assessment and Intervention

Mary Ann Dutton, PhD

The book spells out in practical, concrete terms what it really means to place the pathology outside the battered woman. The novelty in this approach lies in the implications for practice: battered women are not "sick"— they are in a "sick" situation.

"...practical and comprehensive, an excellent guide for clinicians and other interveners.... integrates psychological theory with detailed information on the real-life dimensions of abuse and threat in interpersonal relationships. Her discussion of abused women's posttraumatic responses and the strategies for assessment that form a part of each chapter are particularly valuable."

—Angela Browne, PhD

Partial Contents:

I. Conceptual Framework and Assessment: Women's Response to Battering: A Psychological Model • Understanding the Nature and Pattern of Abusive Behavior • Strategies to Escape, Avoid, and Survive Abuse • Psychological Effects of Abuse • Mediators of the Battered Woman's Response to Abuse

II. Intervention: Framework for Intervention with Victims and Survivors of Domestic Violence • Protective Interventions • Making Choices • Posttraumatic Therapy: Healing the Psychological Effects of Battering • Issues for the Professional Working with Abuse

1992   224pp   0-8261-7130-3   hardcover

536 Broadway, New York, NY 10012-3955 • (212) 431-4370 • Fax (212) 941-7842

🅢 *Springer Publishing Company*

TREATING ATTACHMENT ABUSE
A Compassionate Approach

Steven Stosny, PhD

Attachment abuse can involve both physical and emotional violence between people in close relationships, which includes couples, parents and their children, and adult children and their aging parents, among others. Attachment abusers blame their victims for their own feelings of shame, inadequacy, or inability to love. Dr. Stosny's innovative and integrative approach to the treatment of attachment abuse emphasizes the importance of compassion for both the abused and the abuser. This hands-on manual provides a series of treatment modules designed to teach the perpetrators and the victims how to cope with their feelings and to end attachment abuse.

Contents:

The Role of Attachment in Abuse. Beginnings: Self-Building, Abuse, and Treatment • Attachment • Attachment Abuse: Why We Hurt the Ones We Love • Pathways to Abuse: Deficits in Attachment Skills and Affect-Regulation • A New Response for Clinicians in the Prevention of Emotional Abuse and Violence • Compassion and Therapeutic Morality

Treating Attachment Abuse. The Compassion Workshop • Healing • Dramatic Compassion • Self-Empowerment • Empowerment of Loved Ones • Negotiating Attachment Relationships • Moving Toward the Future

1995   304pp   0-8261-8960-1   hardcover

536 Broadway, New York, NY 10012-3955 • (212) 431-4370 • Fax (212) 941-7842

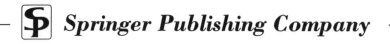

THE PSYCHOLOGY OF SHAME
Theory and Treatment of Shame-Based Syndromes, 2nd Edition

Gershen Kaufman, PhD
Michigan State University

*"This is an extremely thoughtful, creative and ambitious book....
virtually any psychologist who practices or studies psychotherapy
will find this volume useful, enjoyable, and provocative. It addresses
an important but neglected area of human experience. Moreover,
it carefully sets forth its basic assumptions and works from a
theory of human development and experience to create a
comprehensive approach to psychopathology and psychotherapy."*
—Contemporary Psychology

Contents:

1996 368pp 0-8261-6671-7 hardcover

536 Broadway, New York, NY 10012-3955 • (212) 431-4370 • Fax (212) 941-7842

℗ *Springer Publishing Company*

HANDBOOK ON SEXUAL ABUSE OF CHILDREN: Assessment and Treatment Issues

Lenore E. A. Walker, EdD, Editor

This groundbreaking volume presents advances in identification assessment, legal alternatives, and treatment of sexually abused children, as well as their families and the offenders, it presents a range of new treament options including family, community oriented approaches, and individual therapy.

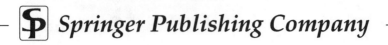

Handbook
on
SEXUAL ABUSE
of
CHILDREN

Lenore E.A. Walker
Ed.D., A.B.P.P.
Editor

Springer Publishing Company

"These papers often challenge traditionally held views; all achieve a high level of clarity and encourage self-examination on the part of the therapist with regard to bias and ignorance..." —Readings

Partial Contents:

- Children as Witnesses: What Do They Remember, *Gail S. Goodman, PhD and Vicki S Helgeson, PhD*

- Legal Issues in Child Sexual Abuse: Criminal Cases and Neglect and Dependency Cases, *Gregory F. Long, JD*

- Incest Investigation and Treatment Planning by Child Protective Services, *Cassie C. Spencer, MSW and Margaret A. Nicholson, MSW*

- New Techniques for Assessment and Evaluation of Child Sexual Abuse Victims: Using Anatomically "Correct" Dolls and Video tape Procedures, *Lenore E.A. Walker, EdD*

- Guidelines for Assessing Sex Offenders, *Kevin McGovern, PhD and James Peters, JD*

- "Taking Care of Me": Preventing Child Sexual Abuse in the Hispanic Community, *Barrie Levy, MSW, LCSW*

Behavioral Science Book Service Selection
1988   480pp   0-8261-5300-3   hard

536 Broadway, New York, NY 10012-3955 • (212) 431-4370 • Fax (212) 941-7842